# Clinical Manual of
# Women's Mental Health

# Clinical Manual of Women's Mental Health

**By**

## Vivien K. Burt, M.D., Ph.D.

Department of Psychiatry and Biobehavioral Sciences,
David Geffen School of Medicine at UCLA, and
Director, Women's Life Center, Neuropsychiatric Institute and Hospital

## Victoria C. Hendrick, M.D.

Associate Professor of Psychiatry,
Department of Psychiatry and Biobehavioral Sciences,
David Geffen School of Medicine at UCLA
and Olive View–UCLA Medical Center

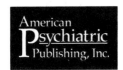

Washington, DC
London, England

Manufactured in the United States of America on acid-free paper
09  08  07  06  05    5  4  3  2  1
First Edition

Typeset in AGaramond and Formata.

American Psychiatric Publishing, Inc.
1000 Wilson Boulevard
Arlington, VA 22209-3901
www.appi.org

**Library of Congress Cataloging-in-Publication Data**
Burt, Vivien K., 1944–
   Clinical manual of women's mental health / by Vivien K. Burt, Victoria C. Hendrick.
— 1st ed.
      p. ; cm.
   Includes bibliographical references and index.
   ISBN 1-58562-186-2 (alk. paper)
   1. Women—Mental health. 2. Mental illness—Sex factors. 3. Psychiatry.
   [DNLM: 1. Mental Disorders. 2. Women's Health. WM 140 B973c 2005]
I. Hendrick, Victoria C., 1963– .  II. Title.
   RC451.4.W6B885 2005
   616.89'0082—dc22
                                                                        2004026968

**British Library Cataloguing in Publication Data**
A CIP record is available from the British Library.

*To our ever-increasing supporters,*
*Bob, Josh, Kira, Michel, Sloane,*
*Gabrielle, David, Alex, Tobias, and Leo*


*And of course, to our mothers,*
*Greta and Gale,*
*whose courage, devotion, and love*
*inspired our careers in women's mental health*

# Contents

# Preface

The text of this manual, an update of the second edition of our *Concise Guide to Women's Mental Health,* reflects the latest data on women's mental health. Although every section has been revised, particularly extensive revisions have been made in the sections describing the use of psychiatric medications in pregnant and breast-feeding women, abortion and contraception, and the use of hormones in menopausal women. The book continues to reflect our expanding clinical experiences in the Women's Life Center.

Although we extensively review the use of psychopharmacological agents to treat women with psychiatric illness, we make frequent references to the importance of multidisciplinary, comprehensive treatment. We believe that psychotherapy and careful attention to social needs are integral parts of the treatment regimen for women with psychiatric illness.

As always, we are indebted to our colleagues, Drs. Lori Altshuler and Rita Suri and to the faculty, fellows, and residents of the Women's Life Center. Once again, the support and expertise of Angela Farrell, M.S.W., has been invaluable and is deeply appreciated.

We trust that this manual, like our concise guide, will serve as a resource for clinicians who care for women with psychiatric illness.

*Vivien K. Burt, M.D., Ph.D.*

*Victoria C. Hendrick, M.D.*

# Introduction

Women use more health care services than any other group in the United States. They make more visits to doctors' offices than do men, fill more prescriptions, have more surgeries, occupy more than 60% of all hospital beds, and spend two of every three health care dollars (Collins 1994). Recognizing the underrepresentation of women in major clinical research trials, the National Institutes of Health (NIH) established the Office of Research on Women's Health in 1990. The National Institutes of Health Revitalization Act of 1993 (P.L. 103-43) stipulated that NIH-funded clinical research should address therapeutic efficacy for women and minorities. Since 1993, active trials in gender-specific aspects of mental health have led to a better understanding of the psychiatric disorders to which women are vulnerable. This book is a guide to the assessment and management of psychiatric conditions specific to women.

## Gender Differences in Psychiatric Disorders

Gender differences in the prevalence of psychiatric disorders have long been recognized; the prevalence in women exceeds that in men for a number of disorders (Anderson et al. 2004; Andrade et al. 2003; Garfinkel et al. 1995; Kessler et al. 1994; Rosenthal et al. 1984; Walters and Kendler 1995) (Table 1–1). Gender-related differences exist not only in the lifetime prevalence of psychiatric disorders but also in the expression, comorbidity, and course of many illnesses. For example, depression and dysthymia, both more common in women than in men, are more likely to be accompanied by anxiety disorders in women (Kornstein et al. 2002). Results from the National Comorbidity Survey and the Epidemiologic Catchment Area survey suggest that depressed women may also be more likely than men to experience anxious somatic depression, which is characterized by prominent sleep and appetite disturbances, aches and pains, and anxiety (Silverstein 2002). Women with chronic major depression tend to have a younger age at illness onset, a more extensive family history of mood disorder, poorer social adjustment, and poorer quality of life, compared with chronically depressed men (Kornstein et al. 2000). Although bipolar disorder is about equally prevalent in both genders, women are more prone to rapid mood cycling (Burt and Rasgon 2004). The course of schizophrenia is more favorable in women, who tend to have later onset of the illness, fewer negative symptoms, and better treatment response than do men (Seeman 2000).

Gender differences in psychiatric conditions may be due in part to psychosocial factors. In 2002, about one-fifth (22%) of children lived only with their mothers (Federal Interagency Forum on Child and Family Statistics 2002), and many face daily challenges to fulfill multiple roles and meet conflicting demands. Furthermore, women's traditionally disadvantaged social status, lower wages, and increased vulnerability to sexual and domestic violence may contribute to their higher rates of depressive and anxiety disorders. Biological differences related to gender may also explain some of the differences in psychiatric illnesses between men and women. Research is increasingly revealing that gender differences exist in brain anatomy and that male and female reproductive hormones produce psychoactive effects (Durston et al. 2001; Steiner et al. 2003). The psychoactive effects of estrogen and progesterone have received particular attention. Estrogen's antidopaminergic (Rao and Kolsch 2003) and serotonin-enhancing (Soares et al. 2003) effects and the modulation of γ-aminobutyric acid (GABA) receptors by metabolites of progesterone (Rupprecht 2003) may play a role in psychiatric disorders in women.

**Table 1–1.** Lifetime prevalence of psychiatric disorders in women and men

| Disorder | Prevalence | |
|---|---|---|
| | **Women** | **Men** |
| Depression[a] | 21.3 | 12.7 |
| Dysthymia[a] | 8.0 | 4.8 |
| Bipolar I disorder[b] | 0.9 | 0.7 |
| Bipolar II disorder[b] | 0.5 | 0.4 |
| Seasonal affective disorder[c] | 6.3 | 1.0 |
| Panic disorder[a] | 5.0 | 2.0 |
| Social phobia[a] | 15.5 | 11.1 |
| Generalized anxiety disorder[a] | 6.6 | 3.6 |
| Schizophrenia[b] | 1.7 | 1.2 |
| Alcohol dependence[a] | 8.2 | 20.1 |
| Alcohol abuse without dependence[a] | 6.4 | 12.5 |
| Drug dependence[b] | 5.9 | 9.2 |
| Drug abuse without dependence[b] | 3.5 | 5.4 |
| Anorexia nervosa[d,e] | 0.5 | 0.05 |
| Bulimia[f] | 1.1 | 0.1 |
| Antisocial personality disorder[a] | 1.2 | 5.8 |

[a]Data from Kessler et al. 1994.
[b]Data from Andrade et al. 2003.
[c]Data from Rosenthal et al. 1984.
[d]Data from Walters and Kendler 1995.
[e]Data from Garfinkel 1995.
[f]Data from Garfinkel et al. 1995.

# Gender Differences in Psychopharmacology

Women are more than 50% more likely than men to receive an antidepressant or anxiolytic agent during a medical visit (Simoni-Wastila 1998). Increasing data show that gender differences exist in the pharmacokinetics and pharmacodynamics of medications. Gender differences have been noted in rates of hepatic metabolism, possibly because of estrogen's inhibitory effect on some hepatic microsomal enzymes (Lane et al. 1999; Pollock 1997; Robinson 2002). By delaying gastric emptying time, progesterone may influence drug absorption. Estrogen and progesterone, both of which are highly protein-bound, may compete with psychotropic medications for protein binding sites. Free, unbound levels of medications may thus vary with reproductive hormone levels. However, the net influence of physiological levels of reproductive hormones on drug metabolism is unclear. Because these hormones may induce some steps in hepatic metabolism while inhibiting others (Yonkers and Hamilton 1995), the pharmacological effects of reproductive hormones are complex and poorly understood.

The effect of the menstrual cycle on psychotropic medication levels is unclear, although case reports suggest that levels may vary across the cycle (Conrad and Hamilton 1986; Kimmel et al. 1992). The use of exogenous hormones (e.g., oral contraceptives or hormone therapy) may additionally influence levels of medications. Exogenous estrogen can inhibit oxidative hepatic enzymes, in particular CRP3A4, thus increasing blood levels of drugs that are oxidatively metabolized (e.g., many tricyclic antidepressants, diazepam, clonazepam, chlordiazepoxide) by as much as 30% (Robinson 2002). Estrogen can also induce hepatic conjugative enzymes, thereby potentially increasing the clearance of drugs that are conjugated before elimination by the kidney (e.g., lorazepam, oxazepam, temazepam) (Robinson 2002).

## Laboratory Evaluation: Significant Considerations for Women

Certain laboratory data are important in the assessment of women patients. For example, because thyroid disorders are not uncommon in women, especially those older than age 40 years, a full thyroid panel should be obtained for women who report changes in energy level, weight, or temperature tolerance. For middle-aged women, data on follicle-stimulating hormone (FSH) and estradiol levels may be helpful in identifying perimenopausal and menopausal status. Pregnancy should be ruled out if psychotropic medications are to be initiated, particularly in women who have had unprotected intercourse or who have recently missed a menstrual period. A pregnancy test registers positive 10–14 days after conception. Commercially available pregnancy tests are simple to use and provide results within 5 minutes. They are 98% accurate, whereas blood tests for β-human chorionic gonadotropin (β-HCG) are 99%–100% accurate.

If a woman reports irregular or absent menses, her prolactin level and thyroid-stimulating hormone level should be measured, because both hyperprolactinemia and hypothyroidism may influence menstrual patterns. Women with hyperprolactinemia, a side effect of certain antipsychotic medications, may require endocrinological consultation. For women with a history of an eating disorder, the evaluation should include a physical and dental examination; laboratory tests for electrolytes, blood urea nitrogen, creatinine, calcium, magnesium, phosphorus, amylase, and serum protein levels; tests of liver and thyroid function; a complete blood count; and an electrocardiogram.

## The Psychiatric Assessment of Women

Gender-specific aspects of the psychiatric assessment of women are summarized in Table 1–2. Clinicians should be alert to the elements of the history that are specifically relevant to women patients. For example, it is important to assess the relationship of the patient's symptoms to her menstrual cycle, to inquire about the possibility that she may be pregnant, and to ask about her use of contraception. The use of concomitant medications that may reduce the efficacy of oral contraceptives (e.g., carbamazepine, oxcarbazepine, modafinil, St. John's wort, topiramate) (Doose et al. 2003) should also be explored. The clinician should also ask about the patient's plans regarding pregnancy, because they may influence the choice of treatment (e.g., choosing psychotherapy vs. pharmacotherapy, initiating treatment with a medication for which data on safety during pregnancy are available). When a middle-aged woman reports sleep impairment, it is important to consider that perimenopausal night sweats may be disrupting her sleep. Seasonality of mood symptoms should be explored, because seasonal affective disorder is more common in women than in men. Women who are preoccupied with their weight should be asked about bingeing and purging behaviors, including use of laxatives, diuretics, and appetite suppressants.

**Table 1–2.** Psychiatric assessment of women: clinically significant considerations

| Component | Consideration |
|---|---|
| History of present illness and past psychiatric history | Characterize symptoms in relation to<br>1. A specific phase of the menstrual cycle<br>2. Use of hormonal contraception<br>3. Pregnancy<br>4. The postpartum period<br>5. Breast-feeding or weaning<br>6. Abortion<br>7. Infertility treatment<br>8. Hysterectomy<br>9. Perimenopause |
| Medications | Include exogenous hormones (oral or injectable contraceptives, postmenopausal hormone treatment, fertility medications) and all over-the-counter medications and supplements. |
| Dietary assessment | Rule out ritualistic or restrictive eating patterns, bingeing, self-induced vomiting, and use of diet pills, laxatives, emetics, diuretics. |
| Alcohol and drug use | Rule out covert use, especially of prescription medications. |
| Family psychiatric history | Include history in female family members of premenstrual dysphoric disorder, postpartum mood disorders. |
| Medical history | Rule out autoimmune illnesses (e.g., lupus, thyroiditis, fibromyalgia) that may present with psychiatric symptoms.<br>Rule out history of sexually transmitted disease that may affect current sexual functioning and childbearing capacity. |
| Menstrual history | Rule out pregnancy, menstruation-related symptoms (e.g., bloating, weight gain, cramping, breast tenderness).<br>Rule out perimenopausal symptoms (e.g., irregular menstrual periods, hot flashes). |
| Social and developmental history | Note sexual preference, relationship styles, level of satisfaction with current relationships.<br>Document tendency to take on certain roles in relationships (e.g., caregiver, nurturer, or dependent or helpless role).<br>Note current or past sexual, physical, or emotional abuse. |
| Socioeconomic status | Note level of economic support and ability to meet ongoing financial needs.<br>If patient is a single mother, inquire about child support. |

Because reproduction-related mood symptoms often run in families, a family history regarding premenstrual dysphoric disorder and depression should be obtained. Women with a history of sexually transmitted illnesses may be left with residual anger, guilt, or sadness that may significantly influence their intimate relationships. Also, they may experience recurrent gynecological conditions (e.g., genital warts, genital herpes) that affect their sexual functioning and psychological well-being. Breast surgery and hysterectomy may influence a woman's sense of femininity and sexuality and may affect her relationship with her partner. Alcohol abuse and drug abuse, although less prevalent in women than in men, are significant problems for some women. Women with a history of psychiatric symptoms occurring in relation to a particular reproductive life event (e.g., during use of oral contraceptives, during the premenstrual or postpartum period, or during periods of increased perimenopausal symptoms) may be at risk for developing psychiatric symptoms at future times of hormonal changes (Freeman et al. 2004; Stewart and Boydell 1993).

The treating clinician should also be aware that social roles and pressures may influence a woman's coping capacity and vulnerability to psychopathology. Economic conditions frequently dictate the extent of access to health care in general and to mental health care in particular. The increasing number of female-headed households and the lower salaries for women, compared with men, are two factors related to economic stress in women. Elderly women are particularly affected by economic difficulties. Because they live longer than men, their increased risk of illness further stresses their financial resources (Collins 1994). A woman may need encouragement to discuss strains in her life, such as family or marital conflict, domestic violence, or exhausting caretaking responsibilities, because she may feel guilty or disloyal about voicing her own needs when they conflict with those of family members.

# References

American College of Obstetricians and Gynecologists: Depression in women: ACOG technical bulletin number 182—July 1993. Int J Gyneacol Obstet 43:203–211, 1993

Anderson AE, Yager J: Eating disorders, in Kaplan & Sadock's Comprehensive Textbook of Psychiatry, 8th Edition. Edited by Sadock BJ, Sadock VA. Philadelphia, PA, Lippincott Williams & Wilkins, 2004, pp 2002–2021

Andrade L, Caraveo-Anduaga JJ, Berglund P, et al: The epidemiology of major depressive episodes: results from the International Consortium of Psychiatric Epidemiology (ICPE) Surveys. Int J Methods Psychiatr Res 12:3–21, 2003

Burt VK, Rasgon N: Special considerations in treating bipolar disorder in women. Bipolar Disord 6:2–13, 2004

Collins JB: Women and the health care system, in Women's Health: A Primary Care Clinical Guide. Edited by Youngkin EQ, Davis MS. Norwalk, CT, Appleton & Lange, 1994

Conrad CD, Hamilton JA: Recurrent premenstrual decline in lithium concentration: clinical correlates and treatment implications. J Am Acad Child Psychiatry 25:852–853, 1986

Doose DR, Wang SS, Padmanabhan M, et al: Effect of topiramate or carbamazepine on the pharmacokinetics of an oral contraceptive containing norethindrone and ethinyl estradiol in healthy obese and nonobese female subjects. Epilepsia 44:540–549, 2003

Durston S, Hulshoff Pol HE, Casey BJ, et al: Anatomical MRI of the developing human brain: what have we learned? J Am Acad Child Adolesc Psychiatry 40:1012–1020, 2001

Federal Interagency Forum on Child and Family Statistics: America's Children: Key National Indicators of Well-Being. Washington, DC, U.S. Government Printing Office, 2002, p 7

Freeman EW, Sammel MD, Liu L, et al: Hormones and menopausal status as predictors of depression in women in transition to menopause. Arch Gen Psychiatry 61:62–70, 2004

Garfinkel PE, Lin E, Goering P, et al: Bulimia nervosa in a Canadian community sample: prevalence and comparisons of subgroups. Am J Psychiatry 152:1052–1058, 1995

Kessler RC, McGonagle KA, Zhao S, et al: Lifetime and 12-month prevalence of DSM-III-R psychiatric disorders in the United States: results from the National Comorbidity Survey. Arch Gen Psychiatry 51:8–19, 1994

Kimmel S, Gonsalves L, Youngs D, et al: Fluctuating levels of antidepressants. J Psychosom Obstet Gynaecol 2:109–115, 1992

Kornstein SG, Schatzberg AF, Thase ME, et al: Gender differences in chronic major and double depression. J Affect Disord 60:1–11, 2000

Kornstein SG, Sloan DM, Thase ME: Gender-specific differences in depression and treatment response. Psychopharmacol Bull 36 (4 suppl 3):99–112, 2002

Lane HY, Chang YC, Chang WH, et al: Effects of gender and age on plasma levels of clozapine and its metabolites: analyzed by critical statistics. J Clin Psychiatry 60:36–40, 1999

National Institutes of Health Revitalization Act of 1993, Pub. L. No. 103-43

Pollock BG: Gender differences in psychotropic drug metabolism. Psychopharmacol Bull 33:235–241, 1997

Rao ML, Kolsch H: Effects of estrogen on brain development and neuroprotection—implications for negative symptoms in schizophrenia. Psychoneuroendocrinology 28 (suppl 2):83–96, 2003

Robinson GE: Women and psychopharmacology. Medscape Women's Health eJournal 7:1, 2002

Rosenthal NE, Sack DA, Gillin JC, et al: Seasonal affective disorder: a description of the syndrome and preliminary findings with light therapy. Arch Gen Psychiatry 41:72–80, 1984

Rupprecht R: Neuroactive steroids: mechanisms of action and neuropsychopharmacological properties. Psychoneuroendocrinology 28:139–168, 2003

Seeman MV: Women and schizophrenia. Medscape Women's Health eJournal 5:2, 2000

Silverstein B: Gender differences in the prevalence of somatic versus pure depression: a replication. Am J Psychiatry 159:1051–1052, 2002

Simoni-Wastila L: Gender and psychotropic drug use. Med Care 36:88–94, 1998

Soares CN, Poitras JR, Prouty J: Effect of reproductive hormones and selective estrogen receptor modulators on mood during menopause. Drugs Aging 20:85–100, 2003

Steiner M, Dunn E, Born L: Hormones and mood: from menarche to menopause and beyond. J Affect Disord 74:67–83, 2003

Stewart DE, Boydell KM: Psychologic distress during menopause: associations across the reproductive life cycle. Int J Psychiatry Med 23:157–162, 1993

Walters EE, Kendler KS: Anorexia nervosa and anorexia-like syndromes in a population-based female twin sample. Am J Psychiatry 152:64–71, 1995

Yonkers KA, Hamilton JA: Psychotropic medications, in Review of Psychiatry, Vol. 14. Edited by Oldham JM, Riba MB. Washington, DC, American Psychiatric Press, 1995, pp 307–332

# 2

# Premenstrual Dysphoric Disorder

In DSM-IV-TR (American Psychiatric Association 2000), the diagnosis of premenstrual dysphoric disorder (PMDD) is considered a mood disorder not otherwise specified and replaces the previously named late luteal phase dysphoric disorder. It describes recurrent physical and emotional symptoms that occur in the last week of the menstrual cycle and remit within a day or two after onset of menstruation. PMDD should be differentiated from premenstrual syndrome (PMS), which has milder physical symptoms and involves minor mood changes (Steiner et al. 2003). PMDD is also different from premenstrual magnification (concurrent diagnoses of PMS or PMDD and a major psychiatric or medical condition) and from premenstrual exacerbation of a current psychiatric disorder or medical condition.

The DSM-IV-TR criteria for PMDD are listed in Table 2–1. Because of the poor reliability of retrospective reports, the diagnosis is made prospectively over at least two consecutive menstrual cycles. Nevertheless, in clinical practice, a provisional diagnosis is often made before confirmation through prospective ratings. Prospective ratings are made with a chart such as that shown in Figure 2–1. Up to 80% of women of childbearing age experience some premenstrual symptoms that vary from mild to severe. By using strict

11

**Table 2–1.**   DSM-IV-TR research criteria for premenstrual dysphoric disorder

A.   In most menstrual cycles during the past year, five (or more) of the following symptoms were present for most of the time during the last week of the luteal phase, began to remit within a few days after the onset of the follicular phase, and were absent in the week postmenses, with at least one of the symptoms being either (1), (2), (3), or (4):

    (1) markedly depressed mood, feelings of hopelessness, or self-deprecating thoughts

    (2) marked anxiety, tension, feelings of being "keyed up," or "on edge"

    (3) marked affective lability (e.g., feeling suddenly sad or tearful or increased sensitivity to rejection)

    (4) persistent and marked anger or irritability or increased interpersonal conflicts

    (5) decreased interest in usual activities (e.g., work, school, friends, hobbies)

    (6) subjective sense of difficulty in concentrating

    (7) lethargy, easy fatigability, or marked lack of energy

    (8) marked change in appetite, overeating, or specific food cravings

    (9) hypersomnia or insomnia

    (10) a subjective sense of being overwhelmed or out of control

    (11) other physical symptoms, such as breast tenderness or swelling, headaches, joint or muscle pain, a sensation of "bloating," weight gain

    **Note:**   In menstruating females, the luteal phase corresponds to the period between ovulation and the onset of menses, and the follicular phase begins with menses. In nonmenstruating females (e.g., those who have had a hysterectomy), the timing of luteal and follicular phases may require measurement of circulating reproductive hormones.

B.   The disturbance markedly interferes with work or school or with usual social activities and relationships with others (e.g., avoidance of social activities, decreased productivity and efficiency at work or school).

C.   The disturbance is not merely an exacerbation of the symptoms of another disorder, such as major depressive disorder, panic disorder, dysthymic disorder, or a personality disorder (although it may be superimposed on any of these disorders).

D.   Criteria A, B, and C must be confirmed by prospective daily ratings during at least two consecutive symptomatic cycles. (The diagnosis may be made provisionally prior to this confirmation.)

MONTH: _____

None 0   Mild 1   Moderate 2   Severe 3

1. Circle days of period   2. Chart severity of symptoms as follows:

| SYMPTOMS | 1 | 2 | 3 | 4 | 5 | 6 | 7 | 8 | 9 | 10 | 11 | 12 | 13 | 14 | 15 |
|---|---|---|---|---|---|---|---|---|---|---|---|---|---|---|---|
| | | | | | | | | | | | | | | | |
| | | | | | | | | | | | | | | | |
| | | | | | | | | | | | | | | | |
| | | | | | | | | | | | | | | | |
| | | | | | | | | | | | | | | | |
| | | | | | | | | | | | | | | | |
| | | | | | | | | | | | | | | | |
| | | | | | | | | | | | | | | | |

| SYMPTOMS | 16 | 17 | 18 | 19 | 20 | 21 | 22 | 23 | 24 | 25 | 26 | 27 | 28 | 29 | 30 |
|---|---|---|---|---|---|---|---|---|---|---|---|---|---|---|---|
| | | | | | | | | | | | | | | | |
| | | | | | | | | | | | | | | | |
| | | | | | | | | | | | | | | | |
| | | | | | | | | | | | | | | | |
| | | | | | | | | | | | | | | | |
| | | | | | | | | | | | | | | | |
| | | | | | | | | | | | | | | | |
| | | | | | | | | | | | | | | | |

**Figure 2–1.** Prospective daily rating chart for premenstrual dysphoric disorder.

DSM-IV-TR criteria, it has been estimated that PMDD occurs in 3%–8% of women of reproductive age; however, the prevalence of premenstrual dysphoria that causes clinically significant distress and dysfunction may be as high as 13%–18% (Halbreich et al. 2003).

# Etiology

A number of etiologies have been suggested for PMDD. They include changes in levels of estrogen, progesterone, follicle-stimulating hormone (FSH), luteinizing hormone (LH), cortisol, dihydrotestosterone, thyroid hormones, endogenous opioids, γ-aminobutyric acid (GABA), and serotonin (Schmidt et al. 1998). Although no single etiology has been established for PMDD, fluctuations of normal plasma concentrations of reproductive hormones do appear to produce psychological symptoms in susceptible women (Schmidt et al. 1998). PMDD occurs only in menstruating women and does not occur in prepubertal girls, pregnant women, postpartum women who have not resumed menstruation, and postmenopausal women. One small study revealed that levels of GABA in the occipital cortex declined across the menstrual cycle in healthy women but increased during the follicular phase in women with PMDD (Epperson et al. 2002). It is therefore possible that the pathophysiological processes of PMDD may not be restricted to the late luteal phase of the menstrual cycle.

# Risk Factors

Women with a history of postpartum depression and mood changes induced by oral contraceptives may be at increased risk for PMDD (Burt and Stein 2002). A history of non-reproductive-related clinical depression also appears to be a risk factor, as does a family history of PMDD (Altshuler et al. 1995; Burt and Stein 2002).

# Evaluation

The components of the evaluation for PMDD are listed in Table 2–2. Frequently, women presenting for treatment of what they believe to be PMDD

**Table 2–2.**    Evaluation of premenstrual dysphoric disorder

| Type of evaluation | Components |
| --- | --- |
| Psychiatric evaluation | History of symptoms, including duration, course, precipitating factors, and previous treatments and response<br>Past psychiatric history, particularly of mood disorders<br>History of alcohol and substance abuse |
| Medical evaluation | Medical history, including assessment of endocrine and gynecological disorders (e.g., thyroid abnormalities, endometriosis, fibrocystic breast disease) |
| Laboratory tests | Complete blood count and chemistry panel, including tests of glucose, calcium, and magnesium levels<br>Thyroid function tests |
| Family history | History of premenstrual symptoms, treatment strategies, and outcome in female relatives |
| Medication use | Assessment of medications that may produce psychiatric side effects (e.g., antihypertensive medications, bronchodilators, antiulcer agents, corticosteroids, analgesics, sedatives, decongestants) |
| Nutritional assessment | Assessment of use of caffeine, salt, and alcohol<br>Rule out potential nutritional deficiencies (e.g., vitamin $B_6$, calcium, magnesium) |

have instead another psychiatric disorder, for example, depression, dysthymia, bipolar disorder, or an anxiety disorder, possibly with premenstrual exacerbation (Hendrick et al. 1996). In other cases, women may be experiencing premenstrual magnification (concurrent diagnoses of PMS or PMDD *and* a major psychiatric or medical condition). Examples include women with both bipolar or unipolar depression and PMDD. To screen for other psychiatric disorders, a careful psychiatric history and a prospective evaluation are important. A medical history and a physical examination, including a pelvic examination, are also necessary to rule out disorders that may present with premenstrual symptoms, such as migraine, endometriosis, chronic fatigue syndrome, fibromyalgia, fibrocystic breast disease, irritable bowel syndrome, and systemic lupus erythematosus (see Table 2–3). Although no specific laboratory tests to screen for PMDD exist, laboratory measures can help to exclude other disorders. If a patient reports lethargy or fatigue, thyroid function tests and a complete blood count should be performed to rule out hypothyroidism or anemia. Because PMDD does not occur in women with nonovulatory cycles, a simple at-home urine test to confirm ovulation may be important for women who menstruate irregularly. Prolactin and thyroid studies should be assessed if a patient reports irregular menstrual bleeding or amenorrhea.

Because diets high in caffeine, salt, and alcohol may worsen PMDD, a nutritional assessment can be useful. Women using hormonal contraception who complain of cyclic mood changes are not experiencing PMDD. Nonetheless, they should be evaluated for contraceptive-induced depression or other mood disorders.

Although prospective daily symptom rating is most useful to establish a diagnosis of PMDD, in practice patients tend to be eager for treatment to begin at the very first visit. For this reason, it may be helpful to mail a prospective rating form to a patient before the initial appointment, especially if the patient will experience an entire menstrual cycle between the dates of the initial phone contact and the first office visit. Reviewing the initial rating form with the patient at the first visit may help her understand the usefulness of obtaining temporal confirmation of premenstrual symptoms (Freeman 2003).

**Table 2–3.**   Medical differential diagnosis of premenstrual dysphoric disorder

Endometriosis
Chronic fatigue syndrome
Migraine
Systemic lupus erythematosus
Irritable bowel syndrome
Epilepsy
Fibrocystic breast disease

# Treatment Strategies

## Nonpharmacological Treatments

Reassurance and support should be offered to all women with PMDD. Educating the patient and her family about her premenstrual symptoms can help reduce feelings of shame, guilt, and helplessness. The daily routine of prospective ratings may give a woman a greater sense of predictability and control of her symptoms and may encourage her to rearrange her schedule to minimize stress during the premenstrual week. For women with mild premenstrual symptoms, nonpharmacological interventions may suffice and should be tried before beginning a medication trial (Table 2–4). The patient should be encouraged, for example, to get adequate sleep during her premenstrual week and to minimize her use of caffeine, salt, alcohol, and nicotine. Exercise, relaxation therapy, and cognitive-behavioral therapy may also reduce symptoms (Altshuler et al. 1995; Blake et al. 1998). These nonpharmacological interventions may also be useful in ameliorating premenstrual symptoms while the patient's diagnosis is established through two monthly prospective ratings. If the patient's premenstrual symptoms developed or worsened after initiation of an oral contraceptive, a switch to another preparation or an alternative form of birth control may be helpful.

**Table 2–4.** Nonpharmacological treatment strategies for premenstrual dysphoric disorder

Education, support
Family intervention
Stress reduction
Dietary changes: reduce salt, alcohol, caffeine
Reduce or discontinue nicotine
Cognitive-behavioral approaches
Exercise
Relaxation techniques

## Pharmacological Treatments

A wide variety of pharmacological treatments have been reported to reduce symptoms of PMDD (Table 2–5). Treatments generally use one of three strat-

**Table 2–5.** Pharmacological treatments for premenstrual dysphoric disorder

| Medication | Dosage | When administered |
|---|---|---|
| **Psychotropics** | | |
| Fluoxetine | 20 mg qd | Throughout cycle |
| Sertraline | 50–100 mg qd | Throughout cycle |
| Paroxetine | 10–30 mg qd | Throughout cycle |
| Clomipramine | 25–75 mg qd | Throughout cycle |
| Nortriptyline | 50–100 mg qd | Throughout cycle |
| Nefazodone | 100–600 mg qd | Throughout cycle |
| Dextroamphetamine | 10–20 mg qd | During symptomatic days |
| Alprazolam | 0.25–5 mg qd | During symptomatic days |
| Buspirone | 15–60 mg qd | Throughout cycle or during symptomatic days |
| **Nonpsychotropics** | | |
| Estradiol | | |
| Implants | 50–100 mg subcutaneously | Every 4–7 months |
| Patches | 2 patches at 100 μg | Every 3 days throughout cycle |
| Oral contraceptives: combination agent containing drospirenone (3 mg) and ethinyl estradiol (30 μg) (Yasmin) | 1 tablet daily | 21 days of combined hormone preparation followed by 7 days of inert tablets |
| Gonadotropin-releasing hormone agonist: leuprolide | 3.75 mg intramuscularly | Every 4 weeks |
| Danazol | 200–400 mg | Daily from onset of symptoms to first day of menses |
| **Diuretics** | | |
| Spironolactone | 25 mg qd–qid | During symptomatic days |
| Hydrochlorothiazide | 25–50 mg qd | During symptomatic days |
| Combination agent containing hydrochlorothiazide and triamterene (Dyazide) | 1 capsule | During symptomatic days |

**Table 2–5.** Pharmacological treatments for premenstrual dysphoric disorder *(continued)*

| Medication | Dosage | When administered |
|---|---|---|
| **Prostaglandin inhibitors** | | |
| Ibuprofen | 600 mg bid–tid | During symptomatic days |
| Mefenamic acid | 250–500 mg tid | During symptomatic days |
| Naproxen sodium | 500 mg qd–bid | During symptomatic days |
| **Vitamins/minerals** | | |
| Vitamin E | 400 IU qd | Throughout cycle |
| Pyridoxine (vitamin $B_6$) | 50–100 mg | Throughout cycle |
| Calcium | 500 mg bid | Throughout cycle |
| Magnesium | 360 mg qd–tid | Midcycle to onset of menses |
| **Antihypertensives** | | |
| Clonidine | 17 µg/kg qd | Throughout cycle |
| Atenolol | 50 mg qd | Throughout cycle |
| **Other agents** | | |
| Bromocriptine | 2.5 mg bid-tid | Day 10 to onset of menses |
| Evening primrose oil | 1–4 g qd | Throughout cycle or from midcycle to onset of menses |
| Naltrexone | 25 mg bid | Days 9–18 of cycle |

egies: symptom relief, modification of a possible biochemical imbalance, and suppression of ovulation.

*Psychotropic Treatments*

Several controlled studies showed that the selective serotonin reuptake inhibitors (SSRIs) (e.g., fluoxetine, sertraline, paroxetine, citalopram) at standard dosages are effective for premenstrual dysphoria, irritability, and tension (Cohen et al. 2004; Rapkin 2003; Yonkers et al. 1996; Yonkers et al. 1997). In comparison with tricyclic antidepressants and bupropion, SSRIs produce greater reduction of premenstrual symptoms (Freeman et al. 1999; Pearlstein et al. 1997) and are recognized as first-line treatments for the psychological symptoms of PMDD (Rapkin 2003). Although both continuous and luteal phase dosing have been found to be effective, continuous dosing is preferable if prospective ratings have not been obtained, because this treatment will address mood symptoms comorbid with PMDD that are present in the follicular as well as the luteal phase (Rapkin 2003). For women with premenstrual anxiety and irritability, alprazolam and buspirone are reasonable choices. Alprazolam should be reserved for patients without histories of substance abuse, and its dose should be tapered and discontinued after the onset of menses. Dextroamphetamine has been reported to improve premenstrual lethargy, poor concentration, and increased appetite when used during symptomatic days.

## Hormonal Strategies

Hormonal therapies are based on the premise that premenstrual symptoms result from the endocrine changes of the menstrual cycle. The drop in progesterone during the luteal phase (second half) of the menstrual cycle has been implicated as etiological in PMDD (Figure 2–2). Progesterone supplementation is sometimes used to treat premenstrual symptoms, but double-blind studies failed to show the efficacy of either natural or synthetic progesterone (Altshuler et al. 1995). Estrogen, administered either subcutaneously or transdermally, has been reported to treat premenstrual psychological and physical symptoms effectively (Altshuler et al. 1995). Side effects include nausea, breast tenderness, and weight gain. For reasons that are unclear, orally administered estrogen does not appear to be effective.

Danazol, a synthetic androgen, suppresses the hypothalamic-pituitary-ovarian axis, thus producing an anovulatory state. It has been reported to reduce premenstrual depression, irritability, edema, anxiety, and breast tenderness. Side effects, which are significant, include acne, weight gain, and hirsutism.

Similar symptomatic relief has been reported with gonadotropin-releasing hormone (GnRH) agonists such as leuprolide. Like danazol, GnRH agonists produce anovulation; both danazol and GnRH agonists cause estrogen to fall to menopausal levels, with the accompanying risks of hot flashes, vaginal dryness, headaches, muscle aches, and occasionally depression. Over the long term, use of GnRH agonists can result in osteoporosis. Until more data exist on the safety of these medications in long-term use, they should not be considered first-line treatments for the symptoms of PMDD.

Although oral contraceptives have been used clinically to treat PMS and

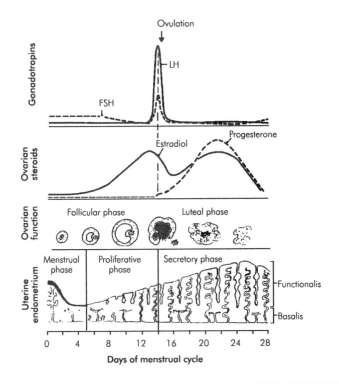

**Figure 2–2.** Hormonal fluctuations across the menstrual cycle.

PMDD, scientific data confirming their effectiveness has been limited and conflicting. Results from a single double-blind, placebo-controlled trial revealed that a unique oral contraceptive (Yasmin) composed of the spironolactone-like progestin drospirenone and ethinyl estradiol had a beneficial effect on symptoms of PMDD, including both physical and mood symptoms (Freeman et al. 2001). Not all results of this study were statistically significant, and larger, more rigorously designed studies are needed to establish the efficacy of this oral contraceptive agent for the treatment of PMDD.

### Vitamins and Minerals

Pyridoxine (vitamin B$_6$), a cofactor in the synthesis of dopamine and serotonin, appears to reduce depression, irritability, fatigue, edema, and headache at a dose of 50–100 mg/day (Wyatt et al. 1999). Patients should be warned not to use pyridoxine excessively, because doses above 100 mg/day have been associated with peripheral neuropathy.

Calcium in doses of 1,200 mg/day has been moderately effective in alleviating premenstrual dysphoric disorder, particularly its physical symptoms, such as edema and pain (Thys-Jacobs 2000). Magnesium and vitamin E have been tried for premenstrual depression, pain, and fatigue. Data from a small controlled study suggested that combining magnesium with vitamin B$_6$ in daily doses of 200 mg and 50 mg, respectively, may produce a modest reduction of mild premenstrual anxiety (De Souza et al. 2000). Although data on their efficacy are mixed, these interventions are worth trying because they are safe and generally well tolerated.

### Diuretics

For women with premenstrual fluid retention, diuretics may be of benefit. Spironolactone and a combination agent containing hydrochlorothiazide and triamterene (Dyazide), help reduce not only premenstrual edema but also premenstrual dysphoria in women who experience diuresis. Hypokalemia, dizziness, and orthostasis are potential side effects. Women who do not experience premenstrual edema do not appear to benefit from diuretics.

### Prostaglandin Inhibitors

Because prostaglandins modulate inflammatory responses and increase pain sensitivity, prostaglandin inhibitors can help reduce pain and swelling. In particular, mefenamic acid and naproxen sodium are effective for premenstrual pelvic pain, cramping, and headache. For maximal efficacy, they should be started before the onset of symptoms (7–10 days before menstruation). The prostaglandin inhibitors do not appear effective, however, for premenstrual mood symptoms.

### Other Agents

A variety of miscellaneous medications have been reported to reduce premenstrual symptoms. The beta-blocker atenolol may improve premenstrual irritability, and the antihypertensive agent clonidine has been reported to relieve premenstrual anxiety, depression, hostility, and irritability. The opiate antagonist naltrexone may reduce general premenstrual symptoms, including irritability, anxiety, depression, lethargy, bloating, and headaches. For premenstrual breast tenderness, the dopamine agonist bromocriptine is helpful and may also reduce premenstrual irritability, depression, and anxiety. Women should be advised to take bromocriptine with food, because it may cause nausea. Evening primrose oil, obtained over the counter in health food stores, has been noted to alleviate premenstrual mood symptoms.

## Approach to Treatment

Before treatment is begun, prospective daily symptom ratings should be obtained to confirm the diagnosis. Psychiatric and medical evaluations should exclude other disorders. Once the diagnosis has been made, simple interventions—for example, exercise, dietary modification, education, and stress reduction—should be encouraged for all patients, even when the decision has been made to initiate pharmacotherapy. In choosing among the various medications, important considerations include the patient's symptom profile and severity, her preference regarding treatment schedule (continuous or during symptomatic periods only), and the medication's side effects and addictive potential.

For patients with mild premenstrual depressive symptoms, vitamins, minerals, evening primrose oil, or a diuretic may be tried. They have the advantage of being well tolerated, and they need to be taken for only part of the cycle.

For patients with more severe premenstrual depression, a psychotropic drug or hormonal agent should be considered. The anxiolytics alprazolam and buspirone are helpful for premenstrual anxiety. To assess for efficacy, a medication trial should extend for a minimum of two or three menstrual cycles. Although more data are needed, oral contraceptives may be used for less severe premenstrual symptoms, particularly if physical symptoms predominate. The oral contraceptive agent that contains a combination of the spironolactone-like progestin drospirenone and ethinyl estradiol may be a good oral-contraceptive choice for treating physical symptoms such as bloating and breast tenderness as well as depressive symptoms. Oral contraceptives have numerous health advantages, such as prevention of bone loss and decreased risks of ovarian and endometrial cancer, abnormal uterine bleeding, and endometriosis (Rapkin 2003).

Medications that suppress ovulation should not be used as first-line options, because little is known about their safety in prolonged use. Because they produce a hypoestrogenic state, they may cause urogenital atrophy and increase the risk of osteoporosis. Although some researchers have suggested that these long-term adverse effects may be mitigated by "add-back" therapy with estrogen and progesterone in doses used for menopausal women, the use of these hormones may induce mood symptoms in women with severe premenstrual mood instability (Rapkin 2003).

For patients with premenstrual symptoms that are refractory to the current treatment strategies, a lasting response has been reported with ovariectomy (Casson 1990). Because this approach produces surgical menopause, estrogen supplementation is necessary. Clearly, this approach is drastic and should not be considered until other treatment strategies have been systematically and exhaustively explored.

Continuation of daily symptom ratings during treatment will allow assessment of symptomatic improvement and may help the patient gain a sense of control over her symptoms by visualizing their timing and predictability.

# References

Altshuler LL, Hendrick V, Parry B: Pharmacological management of premenstrual disorder. Harv Rev Psychiatry 2:233–245, 1995

American Psychiatric Association: Diagnostic and Statistical Manual of Mental Disorders, 4th Edition, Text Revision. Washington, DC, American Psychiatric Association, 2000

Blake F, Salkovskis P, Gath D, et al: Cognitive therapy for premenstrual syndrome: a controlled trial. J Psychosom Res 45:307–318, 1998

Burt VK, Stein K: Epidemiology of depression throughout the female life cycle. J Clin Psychiatry 63 (suppl 7):9–15, 2002

Casson P, Hahn M, Van Vugt DA, et al: Lasting response to ovariectomy in severe intractable premenstrual syndrome. Am J Obstet Gynecol 162:99–105, 1990

Cohen LS, Soares CN, Yonkers KA, et al: Paroxetine controlled release for premenstrual dysphoric disorder: a double-blind, placebo-controlled trial. Psychosom Med 66:707–713, 2004

De Souza MC, Walker AF, Robinson PA, et al: A synergistic effect of daily supplement for 1 month of 200 mg magnesium plus 50 mg of vitamin B6 for the relief of anxiety-related premenstrual symptoms: a randomized, double-blind, cross-over study. J Womens Health Gend Based Med 9:131–139, 2000

Epperson CN, Haga K, Mason GF, et al: Cortical gamma-aminobutyric acid levels across the menstrual cycle in healthy women and those with premenstrual dysphoric disorder: a proton magnetic resonance spectroscopy study. Arch Gen Psychiatry 59:851–858, 2002

Freeman EW: Premenstrual syndrome and premenstrual dysphoric disorder: definitions and diagnosis. Psychoneuroendocrinology 28 (suppl 3):25–37, 2003

Freeman EW, Rickels K, Sondheimer SJ, et al: Differential response to antidepressants in women with premenstrual syndrome/premenstrual dysphoric disorder: a randomized controlled trial. Arch Gen Psychiatry 56:932–939, 1999

Freeman EW, Kroll R, Rapkin A, et al: Evaluation of a unique oral contraceptive in the treatment of premenstrual dysphoric disorder. J Womens Health Gend Based Med 10:561–569, 2001

Halbreich U, Borenstein J, Pearlstein T, et al: The prevalence, impairment, impact, and burden of premenstrual dysphoric disorder (PMS/PMDD). Psychoneuroendrcrinology 28 (suppl 3):1–23, 2003

Hendrick V, Altshuler LL, Burt VK: Course of psychiatric disorders across the menstrual cycle. Harv Rev Psychiatry 4:200–207, 1996

Pearlstein TB, Stone AB, Lund SA, et al: Comparison of fluoxetine, bupropion, and placebo in the treatment of premenstrual dysphoric disorder. J Clin Psychopharmacol 17:261–266, 1997

Rapkin A: A review of treatment of premenstrual syndrome and premenstrual dysphoric disorder. Psychoneuroendocrinology 28 (suppl 3):39–53, 2003

Schmidt PJ, Nieman LK, Danaceau MA, et al: Differential behavioral effects of gonadal steroids in women with and those without premenstrual syndrome. N Engl J Med 338:209–216, 1998

Steiner M, Dunn E, Born L: Hormones and mood: from menarche to menopause and beyond. J Affect Disord 74:67–83, 2003

Thys-Jacobs S: Micronutrients and the premenstrual syndrome: the case for calcium. J Am Coll Nutr 19:220–227, 2000

Wyatt KM, Dimmock PW, Jones PW, et al: Efficacy of vitamin B-6 in the treatment of premenstrual syndrome: systematic review. BMJ 318:1375–1381, 1999

Yonkers KA, Gullion C, Williams A, et al: Paroxetine as a treatment for premenstrual dysphoric disorder. J Clin Psychopharmacol 16:3–8, 1996

Yonkers KA, Halbreich U, Freeman E, et al: Symptomatic improvement of premenstrual dysphoric disorder with sertraline treatment: a randomized controlled trial. JAMA 278:983–988, 1997

# 3

# Hormonal Contraception and Effects on Mood

## Hormonal Contraception

The birth control pill is a popular form of contraception for women. Despite the fact that oral contraceptives are easy to use and when taken as prescribed have an efficacy rate of approximately 99% (Table 3–1), nearly 50% of oral contraceptive users miss one or more pills per cycle, and 22% miss two or more (Rosenberg et al. 1998). It is therefore not surprising that approximately 50% of pregnancies are unplanned, and up to 53% of unplanned pregnancies occur among women who are actively attempting contraception (Cwiak and Zieman 2003).

Advantages of oral contraceptives include regulation of menses and reduction of the risks of endometrial and ovarian cancer, ovarian cysts, ectopic pregnancy, and iron deficiency anemia (Table 3–2). Because of rare risks associated with their use (e.g., thrombovascular disease, hepatic tumors), oral contraceptives are contraindicated in women with certain conditions (Table 3–3). The large variety of formulations currently on the market can be classified into two main categories: combination pills (combining an estrogen and a progestin) and agents containing progestin only (Burkman 2001). Combination pills are further categorized as monophasic (containing fixed doses of estrogen and progestin throughout the cycle) and as biphasic or triphasic (containing varying doses of hormone at different times of the cycle) (Table 3–4).

**Table 3–1.**   Failure rates of various forms of contraception

| Form of contraception | Failure rate Typical use (%) | Perfect use (%) |
|---|---|---|
| No method | 85 | NA |
| Spermicide alone | 21 | 6 |
| Cervical cap with spermicide | 18 | 11.5 |
| Diaphragm with spermicide | 18 | 6 |
| Condom (male) | 12 | 3 |
| Condom (female) | 21 | 5 |
| Oral contraceptives | | |
| Combined | 3 | 0.1 |
| Progestin only | 0.3–0.7 | 0.5 |
| Medroxyprogesterone acetate (Depo-Provera) | 0.3 | 0.3 |
| Levonorgestrel implants (Norplant) | 0.09 | 0.09 |
| Intrauterine device | | |
| Progesterone T | 2 | 1.5 |
| Copper T 380A | 0.8 | 0.6 |

*Source.*   Choice of contraceptives, 1995.

**Table 3–2.**   Risks and benefits of oral contraceptives

| Increased risk | Decreased risk |
|---|---|
| Thromboembolism[a] | Endometrial cancer |
| Cerebrovascular accidents[a] | Ovarian cancer |
| Hypertension[a] | Pelvic inflammatory disease |
| Gallstones | Fibrocystic breast disease |
| Benign hepatic tumors | Iron deficiency anemia |
| Postpill amenorrhea | |

[a]Primarily in smokers older than 35 years.

**Table 3–3.**   Absolute contraindications to use of oral contraceptives

History of thrombophlebitis or thromboembolic disorder

History of coronary artery disease or myocardial infarction

Known or suspected carcinoma of the breast

Known or suspected estrogen-dependent neoplasia, especially carcinoma of the endometrium

Undiagnosed genital bleeding

Markedly impaired liver function

Smoking, age greater than 35 years, and obesity

Known or suspected pregnancy

Congenital hyperlipidemia (estrogen increases risk of cardiovascular death in these patients)

Obstructive jaundice in pregnancy

*Source.*   Speroff et al. 1999.

Brands of combination pills vary in their estrogenic, progestational, and androgenic activity (Table 3–5). In general, estrogenic side effects include nausea, breast tenderness, cystic breast changes, headaches, elevated blood pressure, and increase in the size of fibroid tissue. Progestational side effects include weight gain, fatigue, decreased libido, and headaches. Androgenic effects include hirsutism, acne, and weight gain.

Extended-cycle oral contraceptive regimens have been developed to reduce the number of menstrual periods. One example is a combination agent containing ethinyl estradiol and the progestin levonorgestrel (Seasonale). A tablet containing the active agent is taken once a day for 84 days, after which inert tablets are taken once daily for 7 days. This regimen allows for withdrawal bleeding approximately every third month (as opposed to monthly). This form of oral contraception is believed to be as safe as the more conventional agents and just as efficacious with regard to preventing conception. Extended-cycle oral contraceptives may be particularly useful for women who use birth control pills to relieve heavy periods or severe menstrual cramps and for women who dislike having their periods every month.

Compared with combination pills, progestin-only pills are less effective and may cause irregular bleeding. However, they are indicated for women

**Table 3–4.** Hormonal forms of contraception

Oral contraceptives

    Combination (i.e., with both an estrogen and a progestin component)

        Monophasic (hormone levels remain steady throughout the pill cycle); examples include Brevicon, Loestrin, Demulen, Seasonale

        Triphasic (hormone levels vary across the pill cycle, to simulate a normal menstrual cycle); examples include Ortho-Novum 7/7/7, Tri-Norinyl, Tri-Levlen

    Progestin only; examples include Ovrette, Nor-QD, Micronor

Hormonal patch

    Combination (applied every week for 3 weeks, with fourth week off to allow for withdrawal period); example is Ortho Evra

Injection

    150-mg medroxyprogesterone acetate injection every 3 months (Depo-Provera)

    Combination (i.e., with both an estrogen and a progestin component); example is Lunelle, administered every 28 ± 5 days

Vaginal ring

    Combination (vaginal ring self-administered every 3 weeks, then removed for 1 week to permit withdrawal period)

Intrauterine hormonal device

    Progestin only; example is Mirena intrauterine device (effective for at least 5 years)

Emergency contraception

    Progestin only; example is Plan-B

    Combination; example is Preven

who are breast-feeding or who have contraindications to estrogens (e.g., hypertension, breast cancer).

A hormonal contraceptive transdermal patch (Ortho Evra) releases a combination of ethinyl estradiol and a progestin daily and is applied weekly for 3 consecutive weeks, followed by a patch-free week to allow for withdrawal bleeding. The overall failure rate for this method is much lower than with oral contraception, in large part because compliance is substantially higher among patch users than among users of oral contraceptives (89% vs. 79%) (Cwiak and Zieman 2003).

Two long-acting hormonal forms of contraception, levonorgestrel implants (Norplant) and medroxyprogesterone acetate injections (Depo-Provera), have increased in popularity in recent years because of ease of use and reversibility.

**Table 3–5.** Relative estrogenic, progestational, and androgenic activity of some oral contraceptives

| Contraceptive formulation | Estrogenic activity | Progestational activity | Androgenic activity | Monophasic, biphasic, or triphasic |
|---|---|---|---|---|
| Alesse | + | + | + | Mono |
| Brevicon | ++ | + | + | Mono |
| Cyclessa | + | ++ | + | Tri |
| Demulen | + | + | + | Mono |
| Desogen | + | + | +/− | Mono |
| Estrostep | + | + | + | Tri |
| Genora | ++ | ++ | ++ | Mono |
| Jenest | ++ | ++ | ++ | Bi |
| Levlen | + | ++ | ++ | Mono |
| Levlite | + | + | + | Mono |
| Loestrin 1.5/30 | + | +++ | +++ | Mono |
| Loestrin 1/20 | + | ++ | ++ | Mono |
| Lo/Ovral | + | + | ++ | Mono |
| Mircette | + | + | +/− | Bi |
| Modicon | ++ | + | + | Mono |
| Nordette | + | + | + | Mono |
| Ovcon 1/50 | ++ | + | + | Mono |
| Ovral | +++ | +++ | +++ | Mono |
| Orthocept | + | + | +/− | Mono |
| Ortho-Novum 1/35 | ++ | ++ | + | Mono |
| Ortho-Novum 7/7/7 | ++ | + | +/− | Tri |
| Ortho-Tri-Cyclen | ++ | ++ | + | Tri |
| Seasonale | ++ | ++ | ++ | Mono |
| Tri-Levlen | ++ | + | +/− | Tri |
| Triphasil | ++ | + | +/− | Tri |
| Yasmin | + | + | − | Mono |

*Note.* +++ = highest; ++ = high; + = medium; +/− = low; − = very low.

Levonorgestrel implants are subdermal implants that provides up to 5 years of contraception, and medroxyprogesterone acetate is an injectable progestogenic agent administered every 3 months. Side effects of these methods include menstrual irregularities, acne, and weight gain.

Additional forms of contraception include a vaginal ring containing estrogen and progestin (NuvaRing), a diaphragm-like barrier (Lea's Shield), and a long-acting intrauterine device (IUD) coated with a progestin (Mirena IUD).

Two products are available for emergency, or "morning after" contraception in the United States. Because these agents are administered before the actual fertilization of an egg, emergency contraception does not interrupt an established pregnancy and therefore does not constitute abortion. Plan-B, consisting of two pills, each containing the progestin levonorgestrel (0.75 mg), has been viewed as a second chance to avoid pregnancy and is taken within 72 hours after unprotected sex. Only 1.0% of women will become pregnant after one act of unprotected sex when using this method properly. This form of contraception has also been viewed by some as a contraceptive option for women who have sex infrequently. Another product formulated to achieve emergency contraception has been called the Yuzpe regimen, after an approach used first in the 1970s by Yuzpe and associates (Creinin 1997). This treatment (Preven) comprises a four-pill combined hormonal regimen. Two pills are taken as soon as possible after unprotected sex, and another two pills are taken within 12 hours. The risk of pregnancy is reduced to about 2%, as compared to about 8% in the absence of treatment.

Emergency contraception may also be achieved by using pills from a package of combination birth control pills that contain the progestin norgestrel; each dose must contain 1.0 mg of norgestrel or 0.5 mg of its active isomer levonorgestrol, along with 100 μg of ethinyl estradiol. Depending on the brand of pill, two to five pills are required per dose.

Side effects of nausea may occur with both forms of emergency contraception but are much less common with Plan-B (22% versus 50%). There is much controversy regarding the availability of agents specifically designed to achieve emergency contraception. Despite the recommendation of the American College of Obstetricians and Gynecologists that emergency contraceptives be available over the counter to all women, as of this writing these agents are available only by prescription. In the meantime, it has been suggested that emergency contraception should be prescribed by physicians in advance of need (Westhoff 2003).

# Effects of Hormonal Contraception on Mood

For most women, oral contraceptives do not appear to produce negative mood changes (Yonkers and Bradshaw 1999). In fact, compared to nonusers, users of oral contraceptives have been reported to experience less variability in mood across the entire menstrual cycle and less negative mood during menstruation (Oinonen and Mazmanian 2002). However, certain women do appear at risk for negative mood changes related to oral contraception, including women with a history of depression or other psychiatric symptoms, dysmenorrhea, premenstrual mood symptoms, or pregnancy-related mood symptoms; women with a family history of mood complaints related to oral contraception; and women who are in the postpartum period (Oinonen and Mazmanian 2002). Triphasic preparations—i.e. preparations in which hormone concentrations vary each week—may be particularly likely to induce negative mood changes in these women (Oinonen and Mazmanian 2002).

Independent of their effects on mood, oral contraceptives appear to reduce sexual interest (Graham and Sherwin 1993). Also, contraceptives with high progestational activity (e.g., those containing 1.5 mg norethindrone acetate) may cause fatigue and lethargy. However, somatic symptoms, including premenstrual cramping, bloating, and breast pain, often improve after initiation of oral contraceptives (Graham and Sherwin 1992).

Depot medroxyprogesterone acetate (Depo-Provera) and levonorgestrel implants (Norplant) have been reported anecdotally to cause negative mood symptoms, but studies assessing their effects on mood have found little evidence that they cause depression (Kaunitz 1999; Westhoff et al. 1995).

In conclusion, most women can be reassured that the use of hormonal contraception is unlikely to produce negative mood symptoms. Women with a history of premenstrual mood instability, however, should be warned about the possibility of contraceptive-induced dysphoria. Switching to another hormonal contraceptive or to an alternative method of birth control may lead to resolution of the mood symptoms.

## Drug Interactions Between Hormonal Contraceptives and Other Medications

It is important to keep in mind that hormonal contraceptives can be rendered ineffective by the concomitant use of medications that increase their metabolism. These medications include carbamazepine, oxcarbazepine, topiramate, modafinil, and St. John's wort (Doose et al. 2003). Women should be encouraged to use a high-potency oral contraceptive (i.e., one containing at least 50 μg/day of estradiol) or an alternative method of contraception while taking these medications. Also, one small study reported that estrogen-containing hormonal contraceptives reduced lamotrigine levels by 40%–60% (Sabers et al. 2001), possibly as a result of estrogen's induction of hepatic conjugative enzymes. This induction can also substantially affect levels of other medications that are conjugated before elimination by the kidney, including lorazepam, oxazepam, and temazepam.

## References

Burkman RT: Oral contraceptives: current status. Clin Obstet Gynecol 44:62–72, 2001

Choice of contraceptives. The Medical Letter 37:9–10, 1995

Creinin MD: A reassessment of efficacy of the Yuzpe regimen of emergency contraception. Hum Reprod 12:496–498, 1997

Cwiak C, Zieman M: New methods in contraception: a review of their advantages and disadvantages. Women's Health in Primary Care 6:473–478, 2003

Doose DR, Wang SS, Padmanabhan M, et al: Effect of topiramate or carbamazepine on the pharmacokinetics of an oral contraceptive containing norethindrone and ethinyl estradiol in healthy obese and nonobese female subjects. Epilepsia 44:540–549, 2003

Graham CA, Sherwin BB: A prospective treatment study of premenstrual symptoms using a triphasic oral contraceptive. J Psychosom Res 36:257–266, 1992

Graham CA, Sherwin BB: The relationship between mood and sexuality in women using an oral contraceptive as a treatment for premenstrual symptoms. Psychoneuroendocrinology 18:273–281, 1993

Kaunitz AM: Long-acting hormonal contraception: assessing impact on bone density, weight, and mood. Int J Fertil Womens Med 44:110–117, 1999

Oinonen KA, Mazmanian D: To what extent do oral contraceptives influence mood and affect? J Affect Disord 70:229–240, 2002

Rosenberg MJ, Waugh MS, Burnhill MS: Compliance, counseling and satisfaction with oral contraceptives: a prospective evaluation. Fam Plann Perspect 30:89–92,104, 1998

Sabers A, Buchholt JM, Uldall P, et al: Lamotrigine plasma levels reduced by oral contraceptives. Epilepsy Res 47:151–154, 2001

Speroff L, Glass RH, Kase NG: Clinical Gynecologic Endocrinology and Infertility, 6th Edition. Baltimore, MD, Williams & Wilkins, 1999

Westhoff C: Emergency contraception. N Engl J Med 349:1830–1835, 2003

Westhoff C, Wieland D, Tiezzi L: Depression in users of depo-medroxyprogesterone acetate. Contraception 51:351–354, 1995

Yonkers KA, Bradshaw KD: Hormone replacement and oral contraceptive therapy: do they induce or treat mood symptoms? in Gender Differences in Mood and Anxiety Disorders. Edited by Leibenluft E. Washington, DC, American Psychiatric Press, 1999, pp 91–135

# 4

# Psychiatric Disorders
# in Pregnancy

$P$sychiatric disorders in women arise most frequently between the ages of 18 and 45 years. Since most psychiatric disorders tend to be either chronic or recurrent, many women of childbearing age experience psychiatric illness. For women with preexisting psychiatric illness, little is known about the influence of pregnancy on the course of psychiatric disorders. Available data suggest, however, that pregnancy is not a time of emotional stability, as has been traditionally thought (Evans et al. 2001). Frequently, women with psychiatric histories or those who are currently experiencing psychiatric symptoms request consultation regarding pharmacological management during a future or current pregnancy (Table 4–1).

**Table 4–1.**   Patients requiring perinatal consultation

Patient who is psychiatrically ill during pregnancy
Patient taking psychotropic medication who discovers she is pregnant
Patient with a history of psychiatric illness who is planning to become pregnant
Patient with a history of psychiatric illness who is pregnant

## General Principles

Psychiatric disorders during pregnancy not only affect the mother's well-being but may also increase the risk for poor pregnancy outcomes. Even after adjustment for sociodemographic and obstetric variables, many studies have linked depressive, anxiety, and psychotic disorders during pregnancy with an increased risk of preeclampsia, placental abnormalities, low birth weight, preterm labor, and fetal distress (Chung et al. 2001; Evans et al. 2001; Federenko and Wadhwa 2004; Jablensky et al. 2005; Kurki et al. 2000; Orr et al. 2002; Steer et al. 1992), although other studies have not found these associations (Andersson et al. 2004; Suri et al. 2004). The poor health behaviors associated with depression and anxiety (e.g., poor nutrition, inadequate health care, and use of alcohol and illicit substances) may explain the links with adverse pregnancy outcomes that have been reported in some studies. Alternatively, these adverse outcomes may result from physiological changes associated with these disorders. For example, high concentrations of stress hormones in the third trimester have been found to significantly predict preterm labor (Federenko and Wadhwa 2004). These considerations must be weighed with the potential risks of prenatal medication exposure in an effort to maintain psychiatric stability in the mother while minimizing risks to the developing fetus (Table 4–2).

## Prepregnancy Counseling

More than half of all pregnancies in the United States are unplanned. It is therefore important when prescribing medications for women of childbearing age to consider that they may be pregnant or may become pregnant while taking the medication. If a medication is recommended for treatment of a woman of childbearing age, it is important to consider its potential risks, in-

**Table 4–2.** Management of psychiatric disorders during pregnancy: general principles

Planned pregnancy allows time to discuss treatment options and to switch, if necessary, to a medication that appears safer in pregnancy.

Goal of pharmacotherapy is not maximum control of symptoms but rather reduction of symptoms that jeopardize the mother or the pregnancy.

Whenever possible, psychotherapy and psychosocial measures should take precedence over pharmacotherapy or electroconvulsive therapy.

All treatment recommendations should be discussed with patient, partner, and obstetrician. All discussions before and during pregnancy should be documented.

cluding teratogenicity, neurobehavioral sequelae, and potential associations with impaired fetal growth and perinatal toxicity. These considerations should be discussed in detail with the patient and her partner. The risks of a psychiatric relapse during pregnancy also should be carefully reviewed.

## Pregnancy Planning

Planning for pregnancy is advisable for women with significant psychiatric histories, even if they are not currently symptomatic or taking medications. The goal should be for patients to become pregnant when they are feeling well and able to handle the physiological and psychological demands of pregnancy and parenthood.

Once a patient has decided she would like to become pregnant, a psychiatric consultation should be arranged for her and her partner. The patient's reproductive status and menstrual pattern should be reviewed to evaluate the impact of her fertility potential on planning for pregnancy. For example, a healthy 25-year-old woman is more likely to become pregnant than a woman who is 40 years old. Thus, although it may be reasonable to taper and discontinue psychiatric medications for a young woman who is attempting to become pregnant, it may be less prudent to do so for an older woman who may not successfully conceive for several months. To reduce the risk of psychiatric relapse in an older woman, it may be best to continue psychiatric medications until she becomes pregnant.

For women who wish to breast-feed, a consideration is that some medications are safer than others when used during nursing. All medications that the patient is currently taking, including over-the-counter drugs, should be noted. The importance of remaining free of illicit drugs, nicotine, and alcohol during the pregnancy should be emphasized. The clinician should carefully review the patient's psychiatric history, particularly during any prior pregnancies or postpartum periods. Current treatment and all viable alternative treatment options should be reviewed to justify the implementation of a regimen that will help maintain psychiatric stability while minimizing risks to the fetus. If the treatment recommendation includes the use of psychotropic medication, the available information regarding possible risks to the fetus should be discussed. Ample time should be allowed for questions and clarification. The patient and her partner should be informed that although the U.S. Food and Drug Administration (FDA) does not endorse any psychiatric medication as safe during pregnancy, both the FDA and the American Medical Association agree that physicians may prescribe medications according to their best knowledge and clinical judgment (Gold 2000). All physicians and health care providers who are involved with the patient should be informed about the diagnosis and the course of treatment.

Documentation should indicate how the physician arrived at the recommendations as well as an analysis of the risks and benefits. The documentation should also include a statement indicating that the patient and her partner have been told and understand the benefits and risks involved in the decision and are in agreement with the plan. Some physicians prefer that the patient and her partner sign a statement confirming their understanding of and agreement with the treatment plan. Progress notes should carefully indicate continued analysis of risks and benefits over the course of the pregnancy (Table 4–3).

## Nonpharmacological Interventions

Women should be advised to discontinue the use of caffeine, nicotine, and alcohol during pregnancy. Although sleep disturbance is common during a normal pregnancy, sleep deprivation exacerbates psychiatric symptoms; therefore, an attempt should be made to maximize the opportunity for adequate rest. Relaxation techniques, cognitive-behavioral therapy, and individual psychotherapy can be very helpful for women with anxiety, and environmental

**Table 4–3.** Guidelines for prepregnancy consultation and planning

Meet with the patient and her partner.

Assess reproductive status and likelihood of becoming pregnant.

Inquire whether the patient plans to breast-feed.

Review current medications.

- Prescriptions
- Over-the-counter medications
- Herbs
- Vitamins
- Supplements

Emphasize the avoidance of

- Alcohol
- Drugs
- Nicotine

Review psychiatric history.

Inquire whether the patient has had any prior pregnancies. Review psychiatric course during

- Pregnancies
- Postpartum periods

Consider all treatment options, including current and alternative treatment modalities.

Discuss risks and benefits of treatment options to the patient and to the fetus.

If medication is recommended, provide the patient and her partner with information about risks to

- The fetus
- The infant (if breast-feeding is planned)

Consult with other caregivers, such as the obstetrician, family doctor, pediatrician, and therapist.

Document the initial discussion, including risk-benefit analysis and the patient's understanding of risks and benefits.

Continue documentation of

- Ongoing risk-benefit analysis
- Condition of the patient throughout pregnancy
- Condition of the patient during the postpartum period

**Table 4–4.** Nonpharmacological treatment interventions for psychiatric disorders during pregnancy

Elimination of caffeine, nicotine, and alcohol

Adequate sleep

Relaxation techniques

Interpersonal psychotherapy

Cognitive-behavioral therapy

Support groups

Education

Conjoint therapy with partner

Reduction of psychosocial stressors

Close communication with obstetrical service

interventions (e.g., household help) may help reduce psychosocial stressors. Interpersonal psychotherapy, which focuses on role transitions, deficits in interpersonal interactions, and role disputes, has been found to be an effective intervention for pregnant women (Spinelli and Endicott 2003). If the relationship between the expectant parents is conflictual, conjoint therapy should be strongly encouraged before the delivery. Peer groups for pregnant women, which are becoming increasingly available, may provide the patient with emotional and practical support (Table 4–4).

## Pharmacological Interventions and Electroconvulsive Therapy

Therapy and supportive psychosocial measures may suffice for some women, but more severely ill patients may require psychopharmacological intervention or electroconvulsive therapy (ECT). The decision to use a psychotropic agent in pregnancy always requires a careful weighing of risks and benefits. Whenever a treatment plan is made, the risk to the mother and to the fetus from both the psychiatric disorder and the treatment regimen should be considered. Discontinuation of medication may result in relapse, putting a psychiatrically ill woman at increased risk for poor nutrition, inadequate prenatal care, and substance abuse. However, whenever possible, psychiatric medications should be avoided during the first 12 weeks of gestation, the time of most active organ development in the fetus (Figure 4–1). For a patient who is psychiatrically stable and likely to remain so even without medications for several months or longer, medications should be tapered or discontinued as soon as she discovers she is pregnant. When medications are used during the first 2 weeks postconception, it is unlikely that the developing embryo will be exposed to them because the uteroplacental circulation has not yet fully formed.

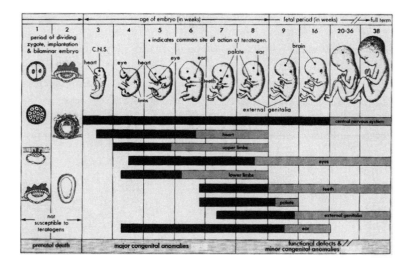

**Figure 4–1.**   Schematic illustration of the critical periods in human development. During the first 2 weeks of life, the embryo is usually not susceptible to teratogens. During these preembryonic stages, a teratogen damages either all or most of the cells, resulting in death, or damages only a few cells, allowing the conceptus to recover and the embryo to develop without birth defects.
**Bar graphs in figure:** *Black,* highly sensitive periods of development when major defects may be produced (e.g., absence of limbs). *Gray,* stages that are less sensitive to teratogens, when minor defects may be induced (e.g., hypoplastic thumbs).
*Source.*   Reprinted from Moore KL, Persaud TVN: *The Developing Human: Clinically Oriented Embryology.* Philadelphia, PA, W. B. Saunders, 1993, p. 156. Used with permission.

When a medication is used during pregnancy, the dose should be maintained at the minimum necessary for control of symptoms. Before administering a psychiatric medication, the clinician should review all available data on the use of the medication during pregnancy with the patient, her obstetrician, and her partner. This review should include the FDA labeling for the medication (Table 4–5) (Physicians' Desk Reference 2004, pp. 217–220). Patients should be advised that the FDA ratings found in the *Physicians' Desk Reference* do not necessarily reflect the standard of care and that the treatment should be based on the latest research findings rather than on these ratings. Patients should also be informed about the limitations of current data, including small sample sizes and confounding factors such as maternal age, diagnosis, and use of additional medications. Moreover, few studies have assessed the potential neurobehavioral sequelae of prenatal medication exposure, a more subtle form of teratogenesis. Toward the end of pregnancy the pediatrician should be provided with information about potential neonatal sequelae of the medications used during pregnancy.

## Use of Psychiatric Medications During Pregnancy

Table 4–6 summarizes the effects of in utero exposure to psychiatric medications.

### Antidepressants

A relatively large literature on the use of tricyclic antidepressants (TCAs) during pregnancy shows that they do not appear to increase the risk for congenital anomalies, even when used during the first trimester (McElhatton et al. 1996). They may, however, produce transient perinatal toxicity or withdrawal symptoms when used near delivery. Symptoms include jitteriness, irritability, lethargy, hypotonia, and anticholinergic effects such as constipation, tachycardia, and urinary retention (McElhatton et al. 1996).

Several recent studies have evaluated the use of the selective serotonin reuptake inhibitors (SSRIs) during pregnancy and have found no evidence of birth defects or miscarriage (Chambers et al. 1996; Cohen et al. 2000; Costei et al. 2002; Ericson et al. 1999; Goldstein 1995; Heikkinen et al. 2002; Hendrick et al. 2003; Kulin et al. 1998; Laine et al. 2003; Nulman et al. 1997; Oberlander et al. 2004; Pastuszak et al. 1993; Simon et al. 1996). However, some studies have reported higher rates of lower birth weight after prenatal

**Table 4–5.** U.S. Food and Drug Administration use-in-pregnancy ratings

| Rating | Interpretation |
|---|---|
| A | Controlled studies show no risk—adequate, well-controlled studies in pregnant women have failed to demonstrate risk to the fetus in any trimester of pregnancy. |
| B | No evidence of risk in humans—adequate, well-controlled studies in pregnant women have not shown increased risk of fetal abnormalities despite adverse findings in animals, or, in the absence of adequate human studies, animal studies show no fetal risk. The chance of fetal harm is remote, but remains a possibility. |
| C | Risk cannot be ruled out—adequate, well-controlled human studies are lacking, and animal studies have shown a risk to the fetus or are lacking as well. There is a chance of fetal harm if the drug is administered during pregnancy, but the potential benefits may outweigh the potential risk. |
| D | Positive evidence of risk—studies in humans, or investigational or postmarketing data, have demonstrated fetal risk. Nevertheless, potential benefits from the use of the drug may outweigh the potential risk. For example, the drug may be acceptable if needed in a life-threatening situation or serious disease for which safer drugs cannot be used or are ineffective. |
| X | Contraindicated in pregnancy—studies in animals or humans, or investigational or postmarketing reports, have demonstrated positive evidence of fetal abnormalities or risk which clearly outweighs any possible benefit to the patient |

*Source.* Reprinted from *Physicians' Desk Reference,* 55th Edition. Montvale, NJ, Medical Economics Company, 2001.

exposure to fluoxetine (Chambers et al. 1996; Hendrick et al. 2003). In one of these studies the low birth weight may have resulted from reduced maternal weight gain rather than the fluoxetine exposure (Chambers et al. 1996). However, the second study found lower birth weight regardless of maternal weight gain, specifically among the infants exposed to relatively high doses of fluoxetine (40–80 mg/day) throughout the pregnancy (Hendrick et al. 2003). It may be that refractory depression during pregnancy, for which the higher doses of antidepressants are prescribed, may be associated with lower birth weight independent of medication exposure.

**Table 4–6.** Summary of effects of in utero exposure to common psychotropic medications

| Medication | Teratogenicity | Potential perinatal effects |
|---|---|---|
| **Antidepressants** | | |
| Tricyclic antidepressants | Appear to be safe: nortriptyline and desipramine preferred. Long-term follow-up to age 7 years suggests no adverse neurobehavioral abnormalities. | Toxicity and withdrawal symptoms have been reported, including lethargy, hypotonia, jitteriness, irritability, anticholinergic effects (e.g., constipation, tachycardia, urinary retention). |
| Selective serotonin reuptake inhibitors | See below for each agent. | For SSRIs in general, some reports have described increased risk of perinatal complications, including jitteriness, tachypnea, respiratory distress, hypoglycemia, poor tone, lower Apgar scores, premature delivery, lower birth weight when used in third trimester. |
| Fluoxetine | No evidence of major congenital anomalies. Long-term follow-up to age 7 years ($N=1,600+$) suggests no adverse neurobehavioral abnormalities. | |
| Sertraline | No evidence of major anomalies ($N=250+$). No long-term neurobehavioral follow-up studies yet. | |

**Table 4–6.**    Summary of effects of in utero exposure to common
psychotropic medications *(continued)*

| Medication | Teratogenicity | Potential perinatal effects |
|---|---|---|
| **Antidepressants** *(continued)* | | |
| Selective serotonin reuptake inhibitors *(continued)* | | |
| Paroxetine | No evidence of major congenital anomalies (*N*=265+). No long-term neurobehavioral follow-up studies yet. | |
| Citalopram | No evidence of major congenital anomalies (*N*=410+). No long-term neurobehavioral follow-up studies yet. | |
| Fluvoxamine | No evidence of major congenital anomalies (*N*=30+). No long-term neurobehavioral follow-up studies yet. | Few data available. |
| Monoamine oxidase inhibitors | Increased rate of congenital anomalies in animal studies. | Contraindicated: potential hypertensive crisis if tocolytic medications are needed. No data available. |
| Trazodone | No evidence of major congenital anomalies (*N*=58). No long-term neurobehavioral follow-up studies yet. | No increased risk of perinatal complications in 58 exposures. |
| Nefazodone | No evidence of major congenital anomalies (*N*=91). No long-term neurobehavioral follow-up studies yet. | No increased risk of perinatal complications in 91 exposures. |

**Table 4–6.**  Summary of effects of in utero exposure to common psychotropic medications *(continued)*

| Medication | Teratogenicity | Potential perinatal effects |
|---|---|---|
| **Antidepressants** *(continued)* | | |
| Venlafaxine | Birth outcomes within expected range in 160 exposures. No evidence of major congenital anomalies. No long-term neurobehavioral follow-up studies yet. | No increased risk of perinatal complications in 160 exposures. |
| Mirtazapine | No evidence of major congenital anomalies but data are limited ($N$=15). | No increased risk of perinatal complications, but data are limited. |
| **Mood stabilizers** | | |
| Lithium | Increased risk for cardiac malformations with first-trimester use. No neurobehavioral sequelae have been noted. | Hypotonia, poor suck reflex, cyanosis, hypoglycemia, neonatal goiter, and diabetes insipidus have been reported. |
| Carbamazepine | Significantly increased risk of neural tube defects with first-trimester exposure. Also, increased risk for developmental delay, craniofacial defects, cardiovascular and urinary abnormalities, and fingernail hypoplasia. | Hypoglycemia, hepatic dysfunction, and bleeding disorders have been reported. |
| Valproate | Significantly increased risk of neural tube defects with first-trimester exposure. Also, increased risk for developmental delay, craniofacial defects, and fingernail hypoplasia. | Hypoglycemia and hepatic dysfunction have been reported. |

**Table 4–6.**  Summary of effects of in utero exposure to common psychotropic medications *(continued)*

| Medication | Teratogenicity | Potential perinatal effects |
|---|---|---|
| **Mood stabilizers** *(continued)* | | |
| Lamotrigine | No evidence of congenital anomalies in more than 970 exposures. | No evidence of perinatal complications. |
| Topiramate | No adverse effects in five exposures. More data are needed. | No adverse effects in five exposures. More data are needed. |
| Oxcarbazepine | No data are available. | No data are available. |
| **Antipsychotic agents** | | |
| Olanzapine | Has not been associated with major congenital anomalies in 150+ exposures. | Has not been associated with perinatal complications. |
| Risperidone | Single case report noted no adverse birth outcomes. | Single case report noted no adverse birth outcomes. |
| Quetiapine | Single case report noted no adverse birth outcomes. | Single case report noted no adverse birth outcomes. |
| Aripiprazole | No data are available. | No data are available. |
| Ziprasidone | No data are available. | No data are available. |
| High-potency antipsychotic agents (e.g., haloperidol, trifluoperazine) | Have not been associated with major congenital anomalies. | Transient perinatal syndrome of motor restlessness, tremor, hypotonia, hyperreflexia, irritability, and poor feeding has been reported in infants exposed near term. |
| Low-potency phenothiazines | May increase risk of nonspecific congenital malformations. No neurobehavioral sequelae have been observed in long-term follow-up of children (to age 5 years). | Transient perinatal syndrome of motor restlessness, tremor, hypotonia, hyperreflexia, irritability, and poor feeding has been reported in infants exposed near term. Neonatal jaundice has also been reported. |

**Table 4–6.**   Summary of effects of in utero exposure to common psychotropic medications *(continued)*

| Medication | Teratogenicity | Potential perinatal effects |
|---|---|---|
| **Anxiolytics** | | |
| Benzodiazepines | Controversial: cohort analysis suggests no increased risk of major congenital anomalies. Case-control data analysis suggests small increased risk of oral clefts. Data on other teratogenic effects are inconclusive. | With regular use in late pregnancy, transient perinatal toxicity syndrome may occur (including neonatal lethargy, hypothermia, hypotonia). Also, infant may experience withdrawal syndrome. |
| Gabapentin | No evidence of congenital anomalies in data from 51 exposures. More data are needed. | No evidence of complications. More data are needed. |
| Zaleplon, zolpidem | No data are available. | No data are available. |
| Buspirone | No data are available. | No data are available. |

Several studies have reported higher rates of perinatal complications and admission to special care nurseries after third-trimester exposure to SSRIs or TCAs (Chambers et al. 1996; Costei et al. 2002; Kallen 2004; Laine et al. 2003). In one study that examined birth outcomes of 209 infants exposed to TCAs during pregnancy and 185 infants exposed to SSRIs, exposure to TCAs was not associated with any significant difference in perinatal outcomes (Simon et al. 1996). However, exposure to SSRIs was associated with a 0.9-week decrease in mean gestational age and, among infants exposed to SSRIs in the third trimester, a 0.29 decrease in mean Apgar score at 5 minutes. This study was based on pharmacy records that indicated drug dispensing but not necessarily actual use of the medications. In another large study, which was based on prospectively recorded information from registry antenatal care records, in utero exposure to antidepressants was associated with an increased risk for preterm birth, low birth weight, and perinatal adverse events, including respiratory distress, low Apgar scores, neonatal convulsions, and hypoglycemia

(Kallen 2004). These adverse events were more prominent with TCA exposure, but they were also found with SSRI exposure.

In April 2004, the U.S. Department of Health and Human Services Center for the Evaluation of Risks to Human Reproduction published an expert panel report on the reproductive and developmental toxicity of fluoxetine (Center for the Evaluation of Risks to Human Reproduction 2004). The panel stated that while third-trimester exposure to fluoxetine may be associated with poor neonatal adaptation, with effects including jitteriness, tachypnea, poor tone, and increased admission to special care nurseries, it is often impossible to differentiate drug-induced adverse effects from those resulting from the psychiatric illness itself. The panel also stated that it is important to weigh possible risks of fluoxetine exposure to a fetus against the known risks associated with untreated psychiatric disease, especially major depression. This advice presumably applies also to the use of other psychiatric medications in pregnancy, especially if these medications are used to stabilize a pregnant woman whose mental condition might compromise her own safety or that of her fetus.

In conclusion, SSRI or TCA use in pregnancy does not appear to produce an increased risk for miscarriage or congenital anomalies. However, the data increasingly appear to show a risk of low birth weight, particularly with prenatal use of fluoxetine. When SSRIs or TCAs are used near term, data also show an increased risk of perinatal complications and somewhat lower Apgar scores. For SSRIs, the severity of these perinatal symptoms appears to correlate with cord-blood concentrations of 5-hydroxyindoleacetic acid, suggesting serotonergic central nervous system effects rather than a withdrawal syndrome (Laine et al. 2003).

Four studies have evaluated the developmental outcomes of children exposed to antidepressants during pregnancy. A recent study reported lower scores on measures of psychomotor development in 31 children of depressed mothers who took SSRIs during pregnancy, compared to 13 unexposed children (Casper et al. 2003). A drawback of the study was the young age of the children, who ranged in age from 6–40 months, as developmental scores in children under age 5 years are generally not predictive of long-term development unless the scores are grossly low. Another study by Nulman et al. (2002), as well as an older study by the same group (Nulman et al. 1997), included children up to age 7 years who were exposed to fluoxetine or to tricyclic antidepressants during pregnancy. These studies did not find differences in temperament, mood, distractibility, behavior, or global IQ in exposed children, compared to unexposed children. The authors reported that maternal depression, however, was associated with less cognitive and language achievement by their children (Nulman et al. 2002). A study of 384 infants exposed to TCAs and SSRIs reported that rates of developmental delay (as assessed from pediatric records) in those children were no different from those in unexposed children (Simon et al. 1996). Women who take SSRI antidepressants during pregnancy should be informed about the sparse data on neurobehavioral outcomes for children exposed to antidepressant medications during pregnancy.

Three studies evaluating venlafaxine ($N$=160), nefazodone ($N$=91), and trazodone ($N$=58) in pregnancy did not find an increased risk of birth defects, miscarriage, or perinatal complications (Einarson et al. 2001, 2003; Yaris et al. 2004). The FDA recently extended its advisory for perinatal complications to include third-trimester use of venlafaxine in addition to SSRIs (http://www.fda.gov/medwatch). The use of bupropion in pregnancy has been associated with a higher risk of spontaneous miscarriage but not with congenital malformations in a study of 99 pregnant women (Einarson et al. personal communication). Although the GlaxoSmithKline Bupropion Pregnancy Registry has not identified an increased risk of congenital malformations among 330 reported exposures, further data are required before a definitive determination can be made about the safety of this agent in pregnancy. Data from two case series of patients who received mirtazapine ($N$=15) reported no congenital anomalies in the infants (Saks 2001; Yaris et al. 2004). Monoamine oxidase inhibitors (MAOIs) should be avoided in pregnancy, because they may produce a hypertensive crisis should tocolytic medications such as terbutaline be used to forestall premature labor. In addition, MAOIs have been associated in animal studies with an increased rate of congenital anomalies.

## Mood Stabilizers

First-trimester use of lithium is associated with a 10- to 20-fold higher incidence of Ebstein's anomaly, a serious series of cardiac defects resulting in displacement of the tricuspid valve into the right ventricle (Briggs et al. 1998; Schou et al. 1973). In some cases, Ebstein's anomaly may be incomplete and asymptomatic, involving some but not all of the defects of this malformation. Although the risk of complete Ebstein's anomaly is 1 per 20,000 in the general population, it appears that first-trimester exposure to lithium increases the risk up to 1 per 1,000 (Altshuler et al. 1996; Cohen et al. 1994). However, the risk may be somewhat higher, as fetal echocardiograms were seldom performed in studies of lithium-exposed pregnancies, and asymptomatic cases may therefore have been missed (Warner 2000). Other cardiac malformations, including coarctation of the aorta and mitral atresia, have also been reported in association with first-trimester use of lithium (Cohen et al. 1994). Lithium use during pregnancy has also been associated with neonatal symptoms, including hypotonia, poor suck reflex, hypoglycemia, and cyanosis (Briggs et al. 1998; Woody et al. 1971). Isolated cases of neonatal goiter and diabetes insipidus have also been reported (Briggs et al. 1998). A 5-year follow-up study of children exposed to lithium in utero, which used data from questionnaires completed by the children's mothers, identified no neurobehavioral sequelae (Schou 1976).

After adjustment for the increased risk of congenital malformations because of epilepsy, the risk for congenital anomalies nevertheless remains elevated in babies born to women treated with valproate or carbamazepine during pregnancy (Altshuler et al. 1996; Dodd and Berk 2004; Iqbal 2000; Matalon et al. 2002). Early first-trimester exposure (i.e., in the first 6 weeks) to valproate is associated with a significant increase in the risk of neural tube defects such as spina bifida, elevating the background risk from 0.03% to 1%–5%. Early first-trimester use of carbamazepine incurs approximately a 1% risk of neural tube defects. Carbamazepine also appears to increase the risk of cardiovascular and urinary tract defects (Matalon et al. 2002; Ornoy and Cohen 1996). Developmental delay, craniofacial defects, and fingernail hypoplasia have been noted with both carbamazepine and valproate (Iqbal 2000; Ornoy and Cohen 1996). The antifolate effects of these medications contribute significantly to their embryotoxicity. Although further data are needed to determine whether high doses of folate reduce the risk of neural tube defects associated with these medications, it is prudent to ensure daily dosing of at least 0.8 mg of folate (i.e., double the recommendation for women who are not at high risk for neural tube defects) by pregnant women exposed to these medications. Unfortunately, folic acid supplements do not appear to diminish the risk of other malformations, such as cardiovascular defects.

Carbamazepine (and other enzyme-inducing antiepileptic drugs, e.g., oxcarbazepine, topiramate) can also produce a deficiency in vitamin K–dependent clotting factors, with a subsequent increased risk of bleeding disorders in the fetus and newborn. Vitamin K supplementation (10 mg/day) should be administered prophylactically to women taking these agents during the last month of pregnancy, and the newborn should receive 1 mg of vitamin K intramuscularly (Iqbal 2000; Morrell 1996). Hypoglycemia and hepatic dysfunction have also been reported in neonates exposed to valproate or carbamazepine during pregnancy (Iqbal 2000; Matalon et al. 2002; Ornoy and Cohen 1996).

In prospective studies of women with epilepsy who are taking lamotrigine, no adverse effects or increased incidence of malformations have been observed in the infants, despite extensive placental passage of the drug (Ohman et al. 2000; Sabers et al. 2004). Data from two pregnancy registries for lamotrigine similarly have indicated no increased risk for congenital anomalies among 637 exposed infants (455 infants exposed to lamotrigine monotherapy and 182 exposed to polytherapy [not including valproate]) (GlaxoSmithKline pregnancy registry data, 2004) and 334 exposed infants (Tennis and Eldridge 2002), respectively. Lamotrigine therefore appears to be a safer choice for pregnant women than valproate, carbamazepine, or lithium. A case series of infants exposed to topiramate (N=5) showed no adverse effects (Ohman et al. 2002). However, more data from human studies are needed before topiramate can be considered safe for use during pregnancy. Although the data from one small study of women with bipolar disorder (N=37) suggested that verapamil is effective in the treatment of mania and mixed states (Wisner et al. 2002), in general the data regarding the efficacy of verapamil for effective treatment of bipolar disorder are equivocal. Therefore, despite its apparent lack of teratogenicity, verapamil is not recommended for use as a primary agent for stabilization of bipolar disorder symptoms during pregnancy.

### Antipsychotic Agents

The low-potency phenothiazines appear to increase the risk of nonspecific congenital anomalies, whereas high-potency antipsychotics—for example, haloperidol and trifluoperazine—have not been associated with a greater rate of fetal anomalies (Altshuler et al. 1996). These data are largely based on the use of low doses of antipsychotic medications for the treatment of nausea and hyperemesis gravidarum. In case reports of clozapine use in pregnancy, infants have been born without malformations (Dickson and Hogg 1998; Stoner et al. 1997), but 8 days after delivery one child experienced a seizure that may have been related to the prenatal clozapine exposure (Stoner et al. 1997). In 23 cases of olanzapine exposure during pregnancy, rates of spontaneous abortion, stillbirth, malformation, and prematurity were within the range of normal historic control rates (Goldstein et al. 2000), and additional case reports noted no adverse birth outcomes (Gentile 2004; Mendhekar et al. 2002). Data from more than 100 exposures are available through September 2000 from the pharmaceutical company pregnancy registry and also show no increased risk of adverse birth outcomes. Single case reports of risperidone and quetiapine use in pregnancy noted no adverse birth outcomes (Ratnayake and Libretto 2002; Tenyi et al. 2002). At the time this chapter was written, no data were available on ziprasidone and aripiprazole use during pregnancy.

A transient perinatal syndrome of motor restlessness, tremor, hypotonia, hyperreflexia, irritability, dyskinesia, and poor feeding has been reported in infants exposed to first-generation antipsychotic agents near term (Altshuler et al. 1996), and neonatal jaundice has been reported after prenatal use of phenothiazine antipsychotics (Tenyi et al. 2002). Although in animals the use of high doses of first-generation antipsychotic agents appears to cause behavioral abnormalities, no neurobehavioral sequelae were noted in a single follow-up study in children with prenatal exposure to these agents (Slone et al. 1977).

### Agents to Treat Antipsychotic-Induced Extrapyramidal Side Effects

Prenatal exposure to the anticholinergic agents trihexyphenidyl and benztropine has been linked to minor congenital malformations, functional bowel obstruction, and urinary retention. Most studies suggest that diphenhydramine does not increase the risk of organ malformation; use of the drug may, however, produce perinatal withdrawal symptoms. Cardiovascular malformations have been noted with exposure to amantadine in utero (Altshuler et al. 1996).

### Benzodiazepines

Data on the use of benzodiazepines during pregnancy are mixed. A recent meta-analysis of cohort studies of benzodiazepine use in pregnancy did not find an association between benzodiazepine use in utero and major malformations (Dolovich et al. 1998). However, a meta-analysis of case-control studies by the same authors did show a small association (relative risk = 1.8) between benzodiazepine use during pregnancy and oral clefts (Dolovich et al. 1998). This risk has been noted particularly for diazepam and alprazolam. Since the background risk of oral clefts is 6 in 10,000, the potential risk of oral clefts is small (less than 12 in 10,000). Nevertheless, it is best to minimize or avoid the use of benzodiazepines during weeks 5–10 of the pregnancy, because the fetal palate forms at this time. Use of benzodiazepines late in the third trimester may be associated with perinatal syndromes, including hypotonicity, withdrawal, failure to feed, apnea, and low Apgar scores (Altshuler et al. 1996; McElhatton 1994; Weinstock et al. 2001). Data are inconclusive on the risk of developmental delay in children exposed in utero to benzodiazepines. Infrequent use of benzodiazepines during pregnancy, however, does not seem to be associated with neonatal difficulties.

*Miscellaneous Agents*

No data from human studies exist for use of buspirone, zolpidem, or zaleplon during pregnancy. Gabapentin was not found to produce an increased incidence of birth defects among 51 exposures reported to a pregnancy drug registry (Montouris 2003).

## Electroconvulsive Therapy

When carried out with a comprehensive treatment team consisting of a psychiatrist, anesthesiologist, and obstetrician, ECT appears to be a safe and effective treatment modality during pregnancy (Altshuler et al. 1996; Miller 1994; Yonkers et al. 2004). It is the treatment of choice when rapid stabilization is essential (e.g., in cases of delusional depression, uncontrollable mania). Preparation should include a pelvic examination, uterine tocodynamometry to rule out uterine contractions, and administration of a nonparticulate antacid such as sodium citrate to reduce the risk of gastric regurgitation, pulmonary aspiration, and aspiration pneumonitis. The patient should be hydrated and adequately oxygenated. During the ECT procedure, for patients in the later stages of pregnancy, the right hip should be elevated to maintain placental perfusion. Use of succinylcholine, a muscle relaxant frequently administered during ECT, appears to be safe during pregnancy. During the procedure, an anticholinergic agent is used to prevent vagal bradycardia and to decrease throat and tracheal secretions. Atropine, sometimes used to prevent vagal bradycardia and decrease respiratory and gastrointestinal secretions, is contraindicated during pregnancy, because it rapidly passes across the placenta, causes fetal tachycardia and variable heart rate, and may mask signs of fetal distress. The anticholinergic agent glycopyrrolate is much less likely to cross the placenta and is therefore a safer alternative. Short-acting barbiturates do not appear to affect the fetus adversely (Miller 1994). External fetal monitoring should continue for several hours after ECT (Table 4–7).

**Table 4–7.**  Electroconvulsive therapy (ECT) for the pregnant patient

Before ECT
  Perform pelvic examination
  Perform uterine tocodynamometry
  Give antacid: sodium citrate
  Begin adequate hydration and continue during procedure
During ECT
  Oxygenate
  Elevate right hip
  Administer succinylcholine for muscle relaxation
  Administer anticholinergic glycopyrrolate
  Administer short-acting barbiturate

# Course and Management of Psychiatric Disorders During Pregnancy

## Depression

In contrast to the common stereotype that pregnancy is a time of emotional well-being, studies have reported that pregnant women experience depression at rates at least as high as nonpregnant women (Bennett et al. 2004; Evans et al. 2001). In these studies, rates of depression have ranged between 12% and 13.5% among pregnant women in the second and third trimesters (Bennett et al. 2004; Evans et al. 2001). Depression may be overlooked in pregnancy because poor sleep, appetite, and energy may be attributed to the somatic experiences of pregnancy rather than to changes in mood.

Risk factors for depression in pregnancy include younger age, lack of social support, living alone, and having more children. Depression during pregnancy triples the risk for postpartum depression and is linked to inadequate prenatal care, poor nutrition, and suicide. Pregnant women with depression are more likely to abuse substances and to deliver babies with fetal distress (Jablensky et al. 2005). As for all psychotropic agents considered for use during pregnancy, antidepressants should be reserved for use only when the risk of not treating an illness in the mother outweighs the possible risk of treatment (Table 4–8).

**Table 4–8.**  Risks associated with psychiatric disorders during pregnancy

Poor prenatal care
Malnutrition
Fetal abuse or neonaticide
Failure to recognize or report signs of labor
Suicide
Poor pregnancy outcomes: low birth weight, preterm delivery, lower Apgar scores
Impulsive behavior (reckless driving, promiscuity)
Use of street drugs, alcohol

When depressive symptoms are mild or moderate, nonpharmacological interventions should be undertaken, particularly in the first trimester. These interventions include psychotherapy, conjoint counseling, modalities to reduce stress, and mobilization of available environmental psychosocial supports. Preliminary data from a small study of 16 pregnant patients with major depression suggested that bright light therapy may produce antidepressant effects (Oren et al. 2002). Because bright light therapy is well tolerated and does not expose the fetus to medication, it may become a promising treatment for depression in pregnant women and certainly should be considered for pregnant women with mild to moderate depression. An additional treatment that may offer an alternative to antidepressants involves the use of omega-3 polyunsaturated fatty acids. These fatty acids not only promote optimal neurological development in the fetus (Willatts 2002) and appear to reduce the risk of preterm labor (Olsen and Secher 2002) but in addition may help treat depression in pregnancy (Chiu et al. 2003).

When symptoms are severe (i.e., the patient is suicidal, psychotic, or not gaining weight), the risk of treatment with medication may be outweighed by the risk of nontreatment. Most data have shown that TCAs, fluoxetine, citalopram, sertraline, and paroxetine do not appear to increase the risks of congenital malformations (Altshuler et al. 1996). Of the TCAs, either nortriptyline or desipramine is best to choose, because these agents produce fewer anticholinergic and hypotensive effects than other TCAs and because blood levels may be followed during pregnancy. Blood levels of medication may drop as pregnancy progresses, possibly because of increased hepatic metabolism, greater volume of distribution, or both. Therefore, it may be necessary to increase antidepressant doses in order to achieve pregravid therapeutic blood levels (Altshuler and Hendrick 1996).

Because poor maternal weight gain has been associated with small-for-gestational-age babies and because depressed pregnant women may not eat properly, it is important that the weight of a pregnant woman who is taking antidepressants be carefully monitored. When needed, ultrasound examinations should be administered to assess whether appropriate gestational development is occurring. Hospitalization and/or ECT should be considered for a suicidal or delusionally depressed pregnant woman.

As was noted earlier in this chapter, a number of studies and reports indicate that third-trimester use of antidepressants may be associated with perinatal toxicity. The decision to treat pregnant women with any psychiatric medication involves a careful risk-benefit analysis. Although controversial, one option, particularly for women on antidepressants who have been psychiatrically stable throughout pregnancy, may be to taper the antidepressant proximate to the expected date of delivery. If this option is chosen, the full dose of antidepressant should be reinstated immediately following delivery, as the postpartum period is a time of high risk in women with histories of depression. Treatment with an antidepressant medication during pregnancy should be instituted only when its benefits are judged to outweigh the possible risks. In many cases, it will not be in the interest of either the mother or the infant to discontinue or reduce the dose of the SSRI in late pregnancy. Discontinuation of antidepressants may precipitate relapse of symptoms and, if done near term, may place the mother at risk during the postpartum period. The adverse effects of undertreated or untreated maternal depression either during pregnancy or the postpartum period should therefore be carefully considered (Koren 2004). In cases in which antidepressant medication has been maintained through pregnancy, the neonate should be monitored carefully, and if there is any indication of adverse effects, the length of hospitalization should be extended beyond the 48 hours (4 days, if delivery was by cesarean section) that is routine in the United States.

## Bipolar Disorder

Data on the course of bipolar disorder in untreated pregnant women are equivocal. One study reported that pregnancy had no effect on the course of bipolar disorder in women who discontinued lithium during the 6 weeks before conception (Viguera et al. 2000). The rate of relapse in these women was no different from the rate in age-matched nonpregnant subjects. In both groups the relapse rate was twice that of the year before treatment was discontinued. The study also found that rapid antepartum discontinuation of lithium resulted in a higher and more rapid postpartum relapse rate than did a slow taper. In another study, pregnancy appeared to protect against decompensation in women with lithium-responsive bipolar I disorder who were not treated with a mood stabilizer during pregnancy (Grof et al. 2000). The few relapses (14% of subjects) occurred in the last 5 weeks of pregnancy. The risk for postpartum decompensation in both studies was high (25%–70%), consistent with previous studies that have shown the postpartum period to be a high-risk time for women with bipolar disorder. In a case series of three women with bipolar disorder who had histories of frequent relapses despite pharmacological treatment, the women experienced euthymia during their pregnancies (Sharma and Persad 1995). Further, hospital admissions for bipolar illness have been reported to drop during pregnancy, compared to nonpregnancy-related admissions. In summary, some women with bipolar disorder may experience stabilization of mood during pregnancy, particularly patients with histories of treatment-responsive illness. However, the postpartum period is a time of substantial risk for decompensation for women with bipolar disorder. More studies are needed to determine whether the reported stabilization, when it occurs, is due to physiological factors related to the pregnancy or to other variables such as increased contact with health practitioners through prenatal visits. Also, future studies should attempt to identify factors that predict a more benign course of illness during pregnancy.

Lithium, carbamazepine, and valproate are associated with increased rates of fetal anomalies when used in the first trimester (Yonkers et al. 2004). Thus, for women with long periods of interepisode well-being, it is worth trying to discontinue these medications before conception. Medications should be tapered gradually (over a period of 2–4 weeks) because abrupt discontinuation of medication increases the risk of relapse (Faedda et al. 1993). When possible, mood stabilizers should be avoided during the first trimester of pregnancy. However, for women with a history of decompensation when they are not taking medication, pharmacotherapy may need to be continued during pregnancy. A relapse of mania poses grave dangers to both the mother and the fetus: poor judgment and impulsive behavior may result in reckless driving, drug abuse, and failure to obtain prenatal care. Dysphoric and psychotic manic episodes are even more hazardous, for they place the patient at risk for suicide and fetal abuse. Because of the more teratogenic potential of carbamazepine and valproate, lithium is a better choice during pregnancy. It should be prescribed in multiple doses per day to avoid exposing the fetus to peak blood levels. Lithium levels should be followed at least monthly because they may drop with the increases in maternal fluid volume and renal clearance. A level II ultrasound should be obtained at week 18 to assess for cardiovascular anomalies. Measurement of nuchal translucency is a new technique that can identify cardiovascular malformations as early as 12 weeks' gestation and is worth considering, keeping in mind that its results are not as accurate as those of the ultrasound at 16–18 weeks. The mother's lithium level should be no higher than 0.9 mEq/L in the 2–4 weeks before the estimated date of delivery to avoid maternal lithium toxicity after the rapid fluid shifts that occur at the time of delivery. Consideration should be given to withholding lithium administration for 1–2 days before a planned delivery (e.g., delivery by cesarean section) or when a woman goes into labor. During labor, maternal lithium concentrations should be carefully monitored, and intravenous fluids should be administered to prevent toxic maternal concentrations, which may occur in association with rapid loss after delivery. Lithium should then be reinstated immediately postpartum. Lamotrigine may also be a reasonable choice to ensure continued mood stability in pregnant women with bipolar disorder. Until further data become available, it is not prudent to use agents such as topiramate or oxcarbazepine for the treatment of bipolar disorder during pregnancy.

ECT is an alternative treatment for women who experience an exacerbation or escalation of symptoms despite other treatment interventions. In cases when carbamazepine or valproate cannot be discontinued in the first trimester, an amniotic α-fetoprotein analysis at gestational week 16 and an ultrasound during weeks 18–22 can be used to screen for neural tube defects. Folate supplementation may reduce the incidence of neural tube defects and should be provided for all women 4 weeks before conception is attempted and throughout the pregnancy.

## Schizophrenia

Schizophrenia has a variable course during pregnancy: some women experience improvement of their condition, whereas the condition of others deteriorates (McNeil et al. 1984a). Older maternal age and fewer physical complications are predictive of a better course (McNeil et al. 1984b). Women with schizophrenia are more likely to experience abruptio placentae, to give birth to small-for-gestational-age babies, and to have children with congenital cardiovascular deformities (Jablensky et al. 2005). Regardless of the course, women with schizophrenia require close follow-up during pregnancy. A relapse or exacerbation of psychosis requires aggressive interventions. Psychosis during pregnancy can lead to fetal abuse or neonaticide, failure to obtain prenatal care, inability to care for oneself, and inability to recognize or report signs of labor. A reduction of psychotic symptoms during pregnancy decreases the likelihood of adverse pregnancy outcomes, such as prematurity, low birth weight, and low Apgar scores. Important interventions include assessment for substance abuse, reduction of psychosocial stressors, and mobilization of family support. Close collaboration with the obstetrical team facilitates the patient's cooperation with necessary medical procedures.

Chronically mentally ill women have a high incidence of losing their children to foster care or adoption. When it appears that the patient may be unable to provide adequate parenting, social service assistance should be requested. Steps can be taken to teach parenting skills, arrange for adequate housing, mobilize family support, and organize financial assistance (Table 4–9).

When possible, antipsychotic agents should be avoided during the first trimester. However, for significantly ill pregnant patients (e.g., patients who experience command hallucinations to harm themselves or the fetus, patients

**Table 4–9.** Important factors to assess in the chronically mentally ill pregnant patient

Social service needs
Custody issues
Parenting skills
Need for financial assistance

unable to care for themselves appropriately because of paranoia or thought disorganization), an antipsychotic may be necessary even in the first trimester. It is advisable to use olanzapine or high-potency first-generation antipsychotics such as haloperidol or trifluoperazine, because more data on use during pregnancy are available for these agents than for other antipsychotic agents (Trixler and Tenyi 1997). When using atypical antipsychotics such as olanzapine during pregnancy, particular care must be given to measurement of serum glucose levels, as these agents may increase the risk of gestational diabetes (Gentile 2004). Doses should be maintained at the minimum necessary for symptom control.

Most agents used to treat extrapyramidal side effects are best avoided during pregnancy because they are associated with major and minor congenital anomalies. However, most studies suggest that diphenhydramine does not increase the risk of congenital malformation. Alternative strategies for patients who experience extrapyramidal symptoms include reduction of the antipsychotic dose and switching to an alternative agent. Women with schizophrenia appear to be at increased risk of having a child with a neural tube defect because of their generally low dietary folate intake and increased likelihood of obesity, two risk factors for neural tube defects (Koren et al. 2002).

A pregnant psychotic woman who refuses prenatal care presents complicated ethical and legal issues. Often the patient can be engaged in treatment through education and support. If the patient's psychosis interferes with her capacity to make informed decisions about her treatment, her psychiatric condition should be treated. If she refuses psychiatric care or is unable to make an informed decision despite receiving psychiatric care, a court order may be necessary to proceed with obstetrical interventions. Psychiatric care can also be enforced if the patient is deemed to be a danger to herself or to others or to be gravely disabled. Whether a pregnant woman who engages in behaviors that are potentially harmful to the fetus can be considered a "danger to others" is a matter of significant legal controversy.

## Anxiety Disorders

Little is known about the course of generalized anxiety disorder during pregnancy. The symptoms of panic disorder improve in some women and worsen in others. Obsessive-compulsive disorder appears to worsen during pregnancy (Abramowitz et al. 2003).

Factors contributing to the course of anxiety disorders during pregnancy include concerns about one's changing roles and responsibilities and the effect of a new child on one's professional, social, and family life. Increased heart rate and respiratory rate, which are physiologically normative in pregnancy, may also contribute to anxiety, as panic attacks may result from catastrophic cognitive reactions to normal physiological events (Cowley and Roy-Byrne 1989). On the other hand, progesterone metabolites, which rise during pregnancy, are active at γ-aminobutyric acid (GABA) receptors and have sedating qualities that may help protect against anxiety attacks

Cognitive-behavioral therapy is an effective treatment for many patients with panic disorder and obsessive-compulsive disorder, and it should be considered as an alternative to medication. Additional nonpharmacological interventions include elimination of caffeine and nicotine, reduction of psychosocial stressors, and initiation of family or couple therapy.

When symptoms are severe and require more aggressive intervention, the TCAs and SSRIs are reasonable treatment options. Benzodiazepines may be necessary initially until the antidepressant medications take effect. Benzodiazepines should be used at the lowest possible dose and if possible should be avoided during the period of oral cleft closure (weeks 5–10). Intermittent use of small doses of benzodiazepines may be necessary at various points during pregnancy. Lorazepam is a reasonable choice, because it has no active metabolites and appears to cross into the placenta at a lower rate than do other benzodiazepines (Whitelaw et al. 1981). Clonazepam is an alternative for patients who require a longer-acting sedative effect. To reduce the risk of toxicity and withdrawal symptoms in the neonate, the use of benzodiazepines should be kept at a minimum near term. To avoid in utero withdrawal, benzodiazepines should be tapered rather than discontinued abruptly during pregnancy.

## Eating Disorders

For many women with bulimia or anorexia, the weight gain of pregnancy represents a failure of the effort to maintain a certain weight and may therefore be difficult to tolerate. Eating disorders during pregnancy increase the risk for complications, including pregnancy-induced hypertension and depression, intrauterine growth retardation, congenital malformations, and failure to thrive (Lacey and Smith 1987) and are associated with an increased likelihood of birth by cesarean section and of postpartum depression (Franko et al. 2001).

Patients with eating disorders should be encouraged to avoid conception until their symptoms have abated. Psychotherapy before and during the pregnancy is important to help reduce the distress these patients may experience because of their changing body shape. Cognitive-behavioral therapy is a particularly effective treatment strategy for bulimia nervosa. When the eating disorder poses a risk to the woman and/or fetus (because of malnutrition, inadequate weight gain, or electrolyte imbalance resulting from vomiting), pharmacotherapy may be necessary. TCAs and SSRIs may be helpful, particularly for bulimia. It should be noted that women with anorexia nervosa have a high incidence of amenorrhea and may have difficulty conceiving.

# Substance Abuse and Pregnancy

Rates of alcohol and substance abuse in women have been rising in the past decade, particularly for cocaine (Greenfield et al. 2003). Approximately 5%–6% of adult American women meet the criteria for alcohol or substance abuse and/or dependence, with women of reproductive age being particularly at risk (Greenfield et al. 2003). Use of alcohol and use of illicit drugs are of great concern during pregnancy because they are associated with an increased incidence of negative obstetrical and perinatal outcomes (Table 4–10).

## Tobacco

Although tobacco is not an illegal drug, its use during pregnancy increases the risk of obstetrical complications and perinatal morbidity. Tobacco has been implicated in spontaneous abortion, placenta previa, and abruptio placentae (Blume and Russell 1993). Cigarette smoking has been linked to intrauterine

**Table 4–10.**   Commonly reported teratogenic effects of abused drugs

| Variable | Opiates | Alcohol | Other sedative-hypnotic drugs | Cocaine | Other stimulants | Hallucinogens | Marijuana | Nicotine |
|---|---|---|---|---|---|---|---|---|
| Specific fetal effects | | | | | | | | |
| Structural nonspecific growth retardation | X | X | — | X | — | — | ? | X |
| Specific dysmorphic effects | — | X | — | X | — | — | — | — |
| Behavioral | X | X | ? | X | X | X | ? | X |
| Neurobiochemical (abstinence syndrome) | X | X | X | — | — | — | — | — |
| Increased fetal and perinatal mortality | X | X | — | X | — | — | — | — |
| Percentage of women reporting use during pregnancy (varies with population) | 5 | >50 | <5 | 20 | <5 | <5 | 5–34 | 50 |

*Note.*   —=effect not reported; ?=data are inconclusive.
*Source.*   Curet and Hsi 2002.

growth retardation and low birth weight and, in some but not all studies, to spontaneous abortion and preterm delivery (Ness et al. 1999). The deficits associated with in utero exposure to tobacco do not appear to be overcome by age 3 years and may include sustained cognitive deficits and behavioral problems such as conduct disorder (Blume and Russell 1993; Fergusson et al. 1998).

## Alcohol

Although the negative effect of alcohol on pregnancy and the developing fetus is due to a combination of pharmacological, lifestyle, and nutritional factors, it is clear that alcohol has direct adverse effects on the obstetrical course and on the developing fetus. Alcohol displaces proteins, vitamins, and essential fats needed for proper fetal development and, with its metabolite acetaldehyde, is directly toxic to fetal cellular growth and metabolism. Alcohol's teratogenic effects produce a spectrum of congenital anomalies ranging from the fetal alcohol syndrome to isolated abnormalities termed *fetal alcohol effects* (McCance-Katz 1991) (Tables 4–11 and 4–12). The incidence of fetal alcohol syndrome is 1–2 per 1,000 live births, and fetal alcohol effects occur at an estimated rate of 3–5 per 1,000 live births. In utero daily exposure to 89 mL or more of alcohol (about three 1-ounce drinks of hard liquor) is associated with a serious risk of fetal alcohol syndrome. Nevertheless, no safe level of alcohol consumption has been established. Women should be encouraged to abstain from alcohol during pregnancy, because even occasional consumption may result in fetal defects (Blume and Russell 1993).

In addition to its teratogenic effects, alcohol has been associated with premature labor, abruptio placentae, stillbirth, and other obstetrical complications. Alcohol may also suppress uterine contractions, thus prolonging labor.

## Cocaine

Adverse effects on the fetus of cocaine use during pregnancy result in part from its acute toxic effects on the mother. Use of cocaine produces maternal hypertension and tachycardia, with subsequent reduction of placental blood flow, placental vasoconstriction, and reduced oxygen transport to the fetus. Cocaine may also have teratogenic potential: exposure to cocaine in utero appears to increase the risk for genitourinary tract malformations (Vidaeff et al.

**Table 4–11.**    Principal features of fetal alcohol syndrome

Structural

  Shortened palpebral fissures (the opening for the eyes between the eyelids)

  Hypoplastic philtrum (dimple of upper lip) and maxilla

  Thinned upper vermilion border of lip

  Retrognathia (backwards displacement of jaw) in infancy

  Micrognathia/prognathia in adolescence (i.e., small or prominent jaw)

  Diminished adipose tissue

Cognitive

  Mild to moderate mental retardation

Developmental

  Poor coordination, hypotonia

  Irritability in infancy

  Attention deficit with hyperactivity in childhood

  Growth retardation

  Height and weight below 95th percentile

*Source.*    McCance-Katz 1991.

**Table 4–12.**    Principal features of fetal alcohol effects

Ptosis (drooping of upper eyelid)

Strabismus (abnormal alignment of one or both eyes)

Epicanthal folds (vertical folds over nasal canthus, i.e., corner of the eye where upper and lower eyelids meet)

Posterior rotation of ears

Prominent lateral palatine (i.e., in the palate) ridges

Cardiac murmurs, atrial septal defects

Labial hypoplasia

Hemangiomas

Abnormal palmar creases

Pectus excavatum (depression of sternum)

*Source.*    McCance-Katz 1991.

2003). However, recent reports have questioned whether the adverse effects of cocaine exposure may be attributable to confounding issues—for example, use of additional drugs or poor diet—rather than to the cocaine (see, e.g.,

Frank et al. 2001; Vidaeff and Mastrobattista 2003). Cocaine's vasoconstrictive effect and its tendency to cause cardiac arrhythmias increase the risk for obstetrical complications, including spontaneous abortion, preterm labor, and abruptio placentae (Vidaeff et al. 2003). Intrauterine growth retardation and fetal distress during labor may occur; neonates may have lower Apgar scores and fetal meconium staining. A prolonged abstinence syndrome, lasting up to 4 months, also occurs in neonates exposed to in utero cocaine. The syndrome is characterized by tremulousness, abnormal motor development, persistence of primitive reflexes, and impaired bonding. Some, but not all studies have reported that extended behavioral abnormalities in babies born to cocaine-abusing mothers may include mood dysfunction and impaired attention. A recent longitudinal, prospective cohort study revealed that prenatal cocaine exposure was not associated with lower verbal or performance IQ scores at age 4 years (Singer et al. 2004). However, prenatal cocaine exposure was associated with selected cognitive impairments and a lower likelihood of achieving an IQ above the normative mean. It is important to note that cocaine-exposed children who lived in a supportive, caregiving home environment had IQ scores similar to those of nonexposed children (Singer et al. 2004).

## Opiates

Heroin use during pregnancy has been associated with an increased incidence of obstetrical complications, including intrauterine growth retardation, premature rupture of membranes, pregnancy-induced hypertension (toxemia of pregnancy), abruptio placentae, neonatal meconium aspiration, maternal and neonatal infections, and stillbirth.

A perinatal withdrawal syndrome associated with heroin use has also been reported, including irritability, decreased feeding, respiratory difficulties, sweating, and tremulousness. This syndrome may be minimized by the use of low-dose methadone and appropriate perinatal care. Opiate-dependent pregnant women may undergo detoxification or may start a methadone maintenance program. Women who are receiving methadone maintenance treatment and who receive proper prenatal care have improved obstetrical outcome, compared with women with untreated opiate use (Blume and Russell 1993).

Other adverse effects associated with in utero exposure to opiates include low birth weight, decreased head circumference, and increased risk of sudden infant death syndrome.

## Cannabis (Marijuana)

Cannabis is fat-soluble and therefore crosses the placenta readily. Once cannabis is in the fetal circulation, its excretion is delayed, and full clearance may not occur for up to 30 days after exposure. Cannabis elevates carbon monoxide levels in the mother and thus decreases fetal oxygenation. Fetal hypoxia also occurs from cannabis-induced maternal tachycardia and hypertension, which reduce placental blood flow.

## Treatment

Goals of the treatment of pregnant substance- and alcohol-abusing women include eliminating alcohol and drug use, treating comorbid medical or psychiatric disorders, assisting the patient safely through the pregnancy, providing assistance for training in parenting skills, and facilitating the patient's continued treatment after pregnancy.

The most important approach to managing the chemically dependent pregnant patient is to provide treatment options in a nonjudgmental and empathic therapeutic setting. Although it is useful to provide the patient with information regarding the harmful effects of alcohol and drugs on obstetrical and fetal outcome, the information should be delivered in the context of managing the substance abuse. Emphasis should be placed on working on a plan to achieve abstinence in order to maximize a return to health for both the mother and the developing baby.

Although pregnancy offers a window of opportunity for treating substance abuse, patients who abuse substances often relapse after pregnancy (at a time when they are responsible for the care of their infants). Rehabilitation, detoxification, and ongoing supportive treatment are necessary to treat the patient during pregnancy and to maximize the opportunity for prolonged success after delivery. A multidimensional approach to treating these patients is essential. The treatment team should include infant and child health care providers, mental health care providers, social service workers, and substance abuse counselors. Attention to practical needs, such as the provision of transportation and child care services, facilitates compliance with a coordinated treatment approach.

Self-help fellowships (Alcoholics Anonymous, Narcotics Anonymous, and Women for Sobriety) are useful. To optimize support for the patient during and after the pregnancy, family members or significant others should be involved. They may benefit from referrals to self-help programs (Al-Anon and Nar-Anon) and to mental health counseling.

The obstetrician and pediatrician should be informed about the nature of the substance use, abuse, or dependence, and all professionals should work closely to support the patient medically, psychiatrically, and obstetrically and ensure the good care of the infant after delivery.

# References

Abramowitz JS, Schwartz SA, Moore KM, et al: Obsessive-compulsive symptoms in pregnancy and the puerperium: a review of the literature. J Anxiety Disord 17:461–478, 2003

Altshuler LL, Hendrick V: Pregnancy and psychotropic medication: changes in blood levels. J Clin Psychopharmacol 16:87–90, 1996

Altshuler LL, Cohen L, Szuba MP, et al: Pharmacologic management of psychiatric illness in pregnancy: dilemmas and guidelines. Am J Psychiatry 153:592–606, 1996

Andersson L, Sundstrom-Poromaa I, Wulff M, et al: Neonatal outcome following maternal antenatal depression and anxiety: a population-based study. Am J Epidemiol 159:872–881, 2004

Bennett HA, Einarson A, Taddio A, et al: Prevalence of depression during pregnancy: systematic review. Obstet Gynecol 103:698–709, 2004

Blume SB, Russell M: Alcohol and substance abuse in the practice of obstetrics and gynecology, in Psychological Aspects of Women's Health Care: The Interface Between Psychiatry and Obstetrics and Gynecology. Edited by Stewart DE, Stotland NL. Washington, DC, American Psychiatric Press, 1993, pp 391–409

Briggs GG, Freeman RK, Yaffe SJ: Drugs in Pregnancy and Lactation, 5th Edition. Baltimore, MD, Williams & Wilkins, 1998, pp 620–625

Casper RC, Fleisher BE, Lee-Ancajas JC, et al: Follow-up of children of depressed mothers exposed or not exposed to antidepressant drugs during pregnancy. J Pediatr 142:402–408, 2003

Center for the Evaluation of Risks to Human Reproduction: NTP-CERHR Expert Panel Report on the Reproductive and Developmental Toxicity of Fluoxetine (NTP-CERHR-Fluoxetine-04). Research Triangle Park, NC, US Department of Health and Human Services, National Toxicology Program, Center for the Evaluation of Risks to Human Reproduction, April 2004

Chambers CD, Johnson KA, Dick LM, et al: Birth outcomes in pregnant women taking fluoxetine. N Engl J Med 335:1010–1015, 1996

Chiu CC, Huang SY, Shen WW, et al: Omega-3 fatty acids for depression in pregnancy (letter). Am J Psychiatry 160:385, 2003

Chung TK, Lau TK, Yip AS, et al: Antepartum depressive symptomatology is associated with adverse obstetric and neonatal outcomes. Psychosom Med 63:830–834, 2001

Cohen LS, Friedman JM, Jefferson JW, et al: A reevaluation of risk of in utero exposure to lithium. JAMA 271:146–150, 1994

Cohen LS, Heller VL, Bailey JW, et al: Birth outcomes following prenatal exposure to fluoxetine. Biol Psychiatry 48:996–1000, 2000

Costei AM, Kozer E, Ho T, et al: Perinatal outcome following third trimester exposure to paroxetine. Arch Pediatr Adolesc Med 156:1129–1132, 2002

Cowley DS, Roy-Byrne RP: Panic disorder during pregnancy. J Psychosom Obstet Gynaecol 10:193–210, 1989

Curet LB, Hsi AC: Drug abuse during pregnancy. Clin Obstet Gynecol 45:73–88, 2002

Dickson RA, Hogg L: Pregnancy of a patient treated with clozapine. Psychiatr Serv 49:1081–1083, 1998

Dodd S, Berk M: The pharmacology of bipolar disorder during pregnancy and breastfeeding. Expert Opin Drug Saf 3:221–229, 2004

Dolovich LR, Addis A, Vaillancourt JMR, et al: Benzodiazepine use in pregnancy and major malformations or oral cleft: meta-analysis of cohort and case-control studies. BMJ 317:839–843, 1998

Einarson A, Fatoye B, Sarkar M, et al: Pregnancy outcome following gestational exposure to venlafaxine: a multicenter prospective controlled study. Am J Psychiatry 158:1728–1730, 2001

Einarson A, Bonari L, Voyer-Lavigne S, et al: A multicentre prospective controlled study to determine the safety of trazodone and nefazodone use during pregnancy. Can J Psychiatry 48:106–110, 2003

Ericson A, Kullen B, Wilholm BE: Delivery outcome after the use of antidepressants in early pregnancy. Eur J Clin Pharmacol 55:503–508, 1999

Evans J, Heron, J, Francomb H, et al: Cohort study of depressed mood during pregnancy and after childbirth. BMJ 323:257–260, 2001

Faedda GL, Tondo L, Baldessarini RJ, et al: Outcome after rapid vs gradual discontinuation of lithium treatment in bipolar disorders. Arch Gen Psychiatry 50:448–455, 1993

Federenko IS, Wadhwa PD: Women's mental health during pregnancy influences fetal and infant developmental and health outcomes. CNS Spectr 9:198–206, 2004

Fergusson DM, Woodward LJ, Horwood LJ: Maternal smoking during pregnancy and psychiatric adjustment in late adolescence. Arch Gen Psychiatry 55:721–727, 1998

Frank DA, Augustyn M, Knight WG, et al: Growth, development and behavior in early childhood following prenatal cocaine exposure: a systematic review. JAMA 285:1613–1625, 2001

Franko DL, Blais MA, Becker AE, et al: Pregnancy complications and neonatal outcomes in women with eating disorders. Am J Psychiatry 158:1461–1466, 2001

Gentile S: Clinical utilization of atypical antipsychotics in pregnancy and lactation. Ann Pharmacother 38:1265–1271, 2004

Gold LH: Use of psychotropic medication during pregnancy: risk management guidelines. Psychiatr Ann 30:421–432, 2000

Goldstein DJ: Effects of third trimester fluoxetine exposure on the newborn. J Clin Psychopharmacol 15:417–420, 1995

Goldstein DJ, Corbin LA, Fung MC: Olanzapine-exposed pregnancies and lactation: early experience. J Clin Psychopharmacol 20:399–403, 2000

Greenfield SF, Manwani SG, Nargiso JE: Epidemiology of substance use disorders in women. Obstet Gynecol Clin North Am 30:413–446, 2003

Grof P, Robbins W, Alda M, et al: Protective effect of pregnancy in women with lithium-responsive bipolar disorder. J Affect Disord 61:31–39, 2000

Heikkinen T, Ekblad U, Kero P, et al: Citalopram in pregnancy and lactation. Clin Pharmacol Ther 72:184–191, 2002

Hendrick V, Smith LM, Suri R, et al: Birth outcomes after prenatal exposure to antidepressant medication. Am J Obstet Gynecol 188:812–815, 2003

Hernandez-Diaz S, Werler MM, Walker AM, et al: Folic acid antagonists during pregnancy and the risk of birth defects. N Engl J Med 343:1608–1614, 2000

Iqbal MM: The effects of valproic acid on fetuses, neonates and nursing infants. Psychiatr Ann 30:221–227, 2000

Jablensky AV, Morgan V, Zubrick SR, et al: Pregnancy, delivery, and neonatal complications in a population cohort of women with schizophrenia and major affective disorders. Am J Psychiatry 162:79–91, 2005

Kallen B: Neonate characteristics after maternal use of antidepressants in late pregnancy. Arch Pediatr Adolesc Med 158:312–316, 2004

Koren G: Discontinuation syndrome following late pregnancy exposure to antidepressants. Arch Pediar Adolesc Med 158:307–308, 2004

Koren G, Cohn T, Chitayat D, et al: Use of atypical antipsychotics during pregnancy and the risk of neural tube defects in infants. Am J Psychiatry 159:136–137, 2002

Kulin NA, Pastuszak A, Sage SR, et al: Pregnancy outcome following maternal use of the new selective serotonin reuptake inhibitors: a prospective controlled multicenter study. JAMA 279:609–610, 1998

Kurki T, Hiilesmaa V, Raitasalo R, et al: Depression and anxiety in early pregnancy and risk for preeclampsia. Obstet Gynecol 95:487–490, 2000

Lacey JH, Smith G: Bulimia nervosa: the impact of pregnancy on mother and baby. Br J Psychiatry 150:777–781, 1987

Laine K, Heikkinen T, Ekblad U, et al: Effects of exposure to selective serotonin reuptake inhibitors during pregnancy on serotonergic symptoms in newborns and cord blood monoamine and prolactin concentrations. Arch Gen Psychiatry 60:720–726, 2003

Matalon S, Schechtman S, Goldzweig G, et al: The teratogenic effect of carbamazepine: a meta-analysis of 1255 exposures. Reprod Toxicol 16:9–17, 2002

McCance-Katz EF: The consequences of maternal substance abuse for the child exposed in utero. Psychosomatics 32:268–274, 1991

McElhatton PR: The effects of benzodiazepine use during pregnancy and lactation. Reprod Toxicol 8:461–475, 1994

McElhatton PR, Garbis HM, Eléfant E, et al: The outcome of pregnancy in 689 women exposed to therapeutic doses of antidepressants: a collaborative study of the European Network of Teratology Information Services (ENTIS). Reprod Toxicol 10:285–294, 1996

McNeil TF, Kaij L, Malmquist-Larsson A: Women with nonorganic psychosis: pregnancy's effect on mental health during pregnancy. Acta Psychiatr Scand 70:140–148, 1984a

McNeil TF, Kaij L, Malmquist-Larsson A: Women with nonorganic psychosis: factors associated with pregnancy's effect on mental health. Acta Psychiatr Scand 70:209–219, 1984b

Mendhekar DN, War L, Sharma JB, et al: Olanzapine and pregnancy. Pharmacopsychiatry 35:122–123, 2002

Miller LJ: Use of electroconvulsive therapy during pregnancy. Hosp Community Psychiatry 45:444–450, 1994

Montouris G: Gabapentin exposure in human pregnancy: results from the Gabapentin Pregnancy Registry. Epilepsy Behav 4:310–317, 2003

Morrell MJ: The new antiepileptic drugs and women: efficacy, reproductive health, pregnancy, and fetal outcome. Epilepsia 37(suppl 6):S34–44, 1996

Ness RB, Grisso JA, Hirschinger N, et al: Cocaine and tobacco use and the risk of spontaneous abortion. N Engl J Med 340:333–339, 1999

Nulman I, Rovet J, Stewart DE, et al: Neurodevelopment of children exposed in utero to antidepressant drugs. N Engl J Med 336:258–262, 1997

Nulman I, Rovet J, Stewart DE, et al: Child development following exposure to tricyclic antidepressants or fluoxetine throughout fetal life: a prospective, controlled study. Am J Psychiatry 159:1889–1895, 2002

Oberlander TF, Misri S, Fitzgerald CE, et al: Pharmacologic factors associated with transient neonatal symptoms following prenatal psychotropic medication exposure. J Clin Psychiatry 65:230–237, 2004

Ohman I, Vitols S, Tomson T: Lamotrigine in pregnancy: pharmacokinetics during delivery, in the neonate, and during lactation. Epilepsia 41:709–713, 2000

Ohman I, Vitols S, Luef G, et al: Topiramate kinetics during delivery, lactation, and in the neonate: preliminary observations. Epilepsia 43:1157–1160, 2002

Olsen SF, Secher NJ: Low consumption of seafood in early pregnancy as a risk factor for preterm delivery: prospective cohort study. BMJ 324:447, 2002

Oren DA, Wisner KL, Spinelli M, et al: An open trial of morning light therapy for treatment of antepartum depression. Am J Psychiatry 159:666–669, 2002

Ornoy A, Cohen E: Outcome of children born to epileptic mothers treated with carbamazepine during pregnancy. Arch Dis Child 75:517–520, 1996

Orr ST, James SA, Blackmore Prince C: Maternal prenatal depressive symptoms and spontaneous preterm births among African-American women in Baltimore, Maryland. Am J Epidemiol 156: 797–802, 2002

Pastuszak A, Schick-Boschetto B, Zuber C, et al: Pregnancy outcome following first-trimester exposure to fluoxetine (Prozac). JAMA 269:2246–2248, 1993

Physicians' Desk Reference, 58th Edition. Montvale, NJ, Medical Economics Company, 2004

Ratnayake T, Libretto SE: No complications with risperidone treatment before and throughout pregnancy and during the nursing period. J Clin Psychiatry 63:76–77, 2002

Sabers A, Dam M, A-Rogvi-Hansen B, et al: Epilepsy and pregnancy: lamotrigine as main drug used. Acta Neurol Scand 109: 9–13, 2004

Saks BR: Mirtazapine: treatment of depression, anxiety, and hyperemesis gravidarum in the pregnant patient: a report of 7 cases. Arch Womens Ment Health 3:165–170, 2001

Schou M, Goldfield MD, Weinstein MR, et al: Lithium and pregnancy, I: report from the Register of Lithium Babies. BMJ 2:135–136, 1973

Schou ML: What happened to the lithium babies: a follow-up study of children born without malformations. Acta Psychiatr Scand 54:193–197, 1976

Sharma V, Persad E: Effect of pregnancy on three patients with bipolar disorder. Ann Clin Psychiatry 7:39–42, 1995

Simon GE, Cunningham ML, Davis RL: Outcomes of prenatal antidepressant exposure. Am J Psychiatry 159:2055–2061, 2002

Singer LT, Minnes S, Short E, et al: Cognitive outcomes of preschool children with prenatal cocaine exposure. JAMA 291:2448–2456, 2004

Slone D, Siskind V, Heinomen OP, et al: Antenatal exposure to the phenothiazines in relation to congenital malformations, perinatal mortality rate, birth weight, and intelligence quotient score. Am J Obstet Gynecol 128:486–488, 1977

Spinelli MG, Endicott J: Controlled clinical trial of interpersonal psychotherapy versus parenting education program for depressed pregnant women. Am J Psychiatry 160:555–562, 2003

Steer RA, Scholl TO, Hediger ML, et al: Self-reported depression and negative pregnancy outcomes. J Clin Epidemiol 45:1093–1099, 1992

Stoner SC, Sommi RW Jr, Marken PA, et al: Clozapine use in two full-term pregnancies (letter). J Clin Psychiatry 58:364–365, 1997

Suri R, Altshuler L, Hendrick V, et al: The impact of depression and fluoxetine treatment on obstetrical outcome. Arch Women Ment Health 7:193–200, 2004

Tennis P, Eldridge RR: Preliminary results on pregnancy outcomes in women using lamotrigine. Epilepsia 43:1161–1167, 2002

Tenyi T, Trixler M, Keresztes Z: Quetiapine and pregnancy (letter). Am J Psychiatry 159:674, 2002

Trixler M, Tenyi T: Antipsychotic use in pregnancy: what are the best treatment options? Drug Saf 16:403–410, 1997

Vidaeff AC, Mastrobattista JM: In utero cocaine exposure: a thorny mix of science and mythology. Am J Perinatol 20:165–172, 2003

Viguera AC, Nonacs R, Cohen LS, et al: Risk of recurrence of bipolar disorder in pregnant and nonpregnant women after discontinuing lithium maintenance. Am J Psychiatry 157:179–184, 2000

Warner JP: Evidence-based psychopharmacology, III: assessing evidence of harm: what are the teratogenic effects of lithium carbonate? J Psychopharmacol 14:77–80, 2000

Weinstock L, Cohen LS, Bailey JW, et al: Obstetrical and neonatal outcome following clonazepam use during pregnancy: a case series. Psychother Psychosom 70:158–162, 2001

Whitelaw AGL, Cummings AJ, McFadyen IR: Effect of maternal lorazepam on the neonate. BMJ 282:1106–1108, 1981

Wisner KL, Peindl K, Perel JM, et al: Verapamil treatment for women with bipolar disorder. Biol Psychiatry 51:745–752, 2002

Willatts P: Long chain polyunsaturated fatty acids improve cognitive development. J Fam Health Care 12(suppl 6):5, 2002

Woody JN, London WL, Wilbanks GD Jr: Lithium toxicity in a newborn. Pediatrics 47:94–96, 1971

Yaris F, Kadioglu M, Kesim M, et al: Newer antidepressants in pregnancy: prospective outcome of a case series. Reprod Toxicol 19:235–238, 2004

Yonkers KA, Wisner KL, Stowe Z, et al: Management of bipolar disorder during pregnancy and the postpartum period. Am J Psychiatry 161:608–620, 2004

# 5

# Postpartum Psychiatric Disorders

For many women, the months after delivery are a time of vulnerability to psychiatric disorders. The incidence of psychiatric conditions, particularly mood disorders, increases significantly in the first 6 months postpartum, compared to other times in a woman's life (Miller 2002). Postpartum mood syndromes are generally classified as postpartum blues (also called maternity blues), postpartum depression, and postpartum psychosis (Table 5–1). Whether these three conditions represent distinct syndromes or rather a continuum is unclear. It is known, however, that they can disrupt family life, have a negative effect on the development of the infant, and increase the risk of subsequent psychopathology in the mother. The postpartum period also represents a time of heightened risk for onset or worsening of panic disorder and obsessive-compulsive disorder (Shear and Mammen 1995).

## Postpartum Blues

The mildest and most common of the postpartum syndromes is postpartum blues (or maternity blues), a transitory state beginning within the first 2–4 days after delivery and lasting no more than 2 weeks. Typical symptoms include tearfulness, mood lability, irritability, and anxiety. The condition occurs

**Table 5–1.**   Postpartum psychiatric disorders: incidence, time course, and clinical features

| Disorder | Incidence (%) | Time course | Clinical features |
|---|---|---|---|
| Postpartum blues | 70–85 | Onset within first postpartum week, abates after 10–14 days | Mood instability, tearfulness, anxiety, insomnia |
| Postpartum depression | 10 | Onset within first postpartum month; duration similar to that of major depressive episode | Depressed mood, guilt, anxiety, fear of harm coming to baby, obsessional features |
| Postpartum psychosis | 0.1–0.2 | Onset within first postpartum month; duration variable— weeks to months | Disorientation, confusion, delusions, hallucinations, often rapid mood cycling |

in up to 85% of all new mothers (O'Hara and Swain 1996) and is thus an expected transient reaction after delivery. Women and their partners benefit from support and reassurance that the symptoms are common and will end soon. Because new mothers are frequently discharged from the hospital on the first or second postpartum day, it may be helpful to provide some information regarding this condition to women before delivery.

## Risk Factors

A history of depression, particularly depression during pregnancy, increases the risk of postpartum blues. A history of premenstrual dysphoric disorder also appears to be a risk factor.

## Treatment

Because postpartum blues are transitory and have no long-term consequences, medical and psychiatric interventions are not necessary. Reassurance, support, and education are enough in most cases. Women should be monitored to ensure that their symptoms do not persist or evolve into postpartum depression.

# Postpartum Depression

Postpartum depression tends to have a later onset than postpartum blues, beginning usually at 2–4 weeks postpartum. Prevalence data suggest a 12%–13% risk of major depression in the postpartum period, a rate equaling that in the general female population (O'Hara and Swain 1996). Nevertheless, postpartum women do appear to have increased rates of depressive symptoms not meeting criteria for major depression (O'Hara 1995). Depressive symptoms occurring during the postpartum period deserve special attention because they cause considerable distress for the patient and her family and tend to be long lasting (Zelkowitz and Milet 2001).

The potential negative consequences of postpartum depression to the emotional and cognitive development of the infant add to the importance of diagnosing and treating this condition (O'Hara and Swain 1996). Postpartum depression increases the risk of negative parenting behaviors and places children at risk for adverse outcomes in social, emotional, and behavioral development (Brennan et al. 2000; Lyons-Ruth et al. 2002). Compared with children of nondepressed mothers, children of depressed mothers have more difficulty with emotional regulation and display more negative affect toward others. Their self-esteem tends to be lower, and they show more aggressive behavior toward their parents and peers, as assessed by evaluations at ages 3–5 years (Sinclair and Murray 1998). They are more prone to helpless behaviors and demonstrate poor social competence, compared with children of nondepressed parents. Early interventions are important, because the degree of risk to children appears related to the duration of the mother's depression (Field et al. 1996). Prompt treatment of maternal depression can significantly reduce adverse consequences to the infant related to that depression, including behavioral problems and patterns of insecure attachment (Cooper and Murray 1997; Grace et al. 2003). Recent research also shows that nursing infants of depressed mothers may gain less weight, compared to infants of nondepressed mothers (Hendrick et al. 2003), possibly because maternal depression may affect a woman's nutrition, breast-feeding habits, or sensitivity to her infant's hunger cries.

Failure to diagnose postpartum depression may arise in part from the focus on the well-being of the baby rather than on that of the mother after delivery. New mothers, sensing societal expectations that they be content and fulfilled, may be reluctant to reveal their feelings. Furthermore, families and physicians may dismiss a woman's symptoms, attributing them solely to the stress of looking after a newborn child.

## Risk Factors

A previous history of major depression is associated with a 24% risk of depression after childbirth (O'Hara 1995). A history of depression occurring during pregnancy is associated with a still higher risk, 35% (O'Hara 1995). Previous postpartum depression is a particularly significant risk factor for recurrence, conferring a recurrence risk of up to 50% (O'Hara 1995). Stressful life events and a lack of support, particularly from the woman's partner, also increase the risk of postpartum depression (Table 5–2). Obstetrical complications and breast-feeding do not appear to be associated with postpartum depression (O'Hara 1995).

**Table 5–2.** Risk factors for postpartum psychiatric disorders

| Disorder | Risk factors |
|---|---|
| Postpartum blues | Depressive symptoms during pregnancy<br>History of depression<br>History of premenstrual dysphoric disorder |
| Postpartum depression | Depression during pregnancy<br>History of depression, especially postpartum depression<br>Dysfunctional marital relationship<br>Inadequate social supports<br>Stressful life events during pregnancy |
| Postpartum psychosis | History of bipolar disorder<br>Primiparity<br>Previous postpartum psychosis |

## Treatment

The most successful treatment strategies are multifactorial. They include education, psychotherapy, group support, referrals to self-help and national organizations (Table 5–3), and conjoint counseling if the relationship with the partner is problematic. Interpersonal therapy and cognitive-behavioral therapy have been found to be effective in treating postpartum depression (Appleby et al. 1997; O'Hara et al. 2000; Segre et al. 2004).

**Table 5–3.**   Treatment options for postpartum psychiatric disorders

| Disorder | Treatment options |
| --- | --- |
| Postpartum blues | Education |
| | Support |
| | Reassurance |
| Postpartum depression | Reduction of psychosocial stressors |
| | Individual and/or group psychotherapy |
| | Antidepressant medications |
| | Electroconvulsive therapy (ECT) |
| | Hospitalization |
| Postpartum psychosis | Hospitalization |
| | Medical workup to rule out organic etiology |
| | Mood stabilizers |
| | Antipsychotics |
| | Antidepressants |
| | Benzodiazepines |
| | ECT |

The patient should be encouraged to obtain support from family and friends for infant care, to get as much sleep and rest as possible, and to reduce her other responsibilities. If possible, the presence of a child care assistant for even part of each day is extremely helpful. Antidepressant medications are often very effective (see, e.g., Cohen et al. 2001). The decision to use medications should include consideration of whether the patient will be breast-feeding (see below). Spouses and partners should be involved in the treatment, because their support is essential for successful management of postpartum depression.

Thyroid function should be evaluated in postpartum women who present with mood or anxiety complaints, as the postpartum period is a time of increased risk for thyroid dysfunction (Stagnaro-Green 2002). In cases of thyroid dysfunction, appropriate treatment is directed at correcting the primary endocrine problem and does not generally involve psychotropic medications.

Women with a history of depression, particularly postpartum depression, are at high risk for recurrence following a subsequent pregnancy. Although the data are conflicting, prophylactic antidepressants (e.g., begun within the first 1–2 days after delivery) merit consideration to reduce the risk of relapse (Wisner and Wheeler 1994; Wisner et al. 2001).

Estrogen has been successfully used to treat postpartum depression in two studies. In the first, a double-blind study of 61 women with major depression that began 3 months postpartum, use of transdermal estrogen led to a rapid improvement in depression ratings, but the depression ratings remained elevated for many women, suggesting that the antidepressant effect was not robust (Gregoire et al. 1996). The second study was an open investigation that included 23 women with major depression occurring in the 6 months after delivery who took sublingual estrogen (Ahokas et al. 2001). After 2 weeks of treatment, 19 of the women experienced a clinical recovery. The use of estrogen, however, is associated with several risks, including endometrial hyperplasia and thromboembolism. It also diminishes the production of breast milk in nursing mothers. Given these considerations and the availability of alternative treatments, estrogen does not appear to have a primary role in the treatment of postpartum depression at this time.

The treatment of postpartum depression with natural progesterone has yet to be evaluated in a clinical trial. Natural progesterone is metabolized into allopregnanolone, a neuroactive steroid that enhances the activity of $\gamma$-aminobutyric acid (GABA) in the central nervous system, producing anxiolytic effects (Rupprecht and Holsboer 1999). Data from carefully controlled studies are needed to determine if natural progesterone has a place in the treatment of postpartum depression with comorbid anxiety. Synthetic progestins, on the other hand, do not help postpartum depression and may, on the contrary, exacerbate the symptoms (Lawrie et al. 2000). Unlike natural progesterone, synthetic progestins (e.g. medroxyprogesterone) are not metabolized into GABAergic neuroactive steroids.

Bright light therapy produced antidepressant effects in two women with postpartum-onset major depression (Corral et al. 2000). Because it is well tolerated and does not produce medication exposure to the nursing infant, bright light therapy may become a promising treatment for postpartum depression. Massage therapy and relaxation training are additional nonpharmacological approaches for postpartum depression that appear to produce more positive mother-infant interactions and better growth and health in the infant (Field et al. 2000).

# Postpartum Psychosis

Postpartum psychosis is an acute, severe illness occurring at a rate of 1–2 per 1,000 births (O'Hara and Swain 1996). Symptoms include lability of mood, severe agitation, confusion, thought disorganization, hallucinations, and sleeplessness. Many researchers believe that postpartum psychosis is a manifestation of bipolar disorder (Chaudron and Pies 2003). After an episode of postpartum psychosis, women are at risk for subsequent nonpostpartum manic-depressive relapses (Rohde and Marneros 1992).

## Risk Factors

A significant risk factor for postpartum psychosis is a history of bipolar disorder, which has been reported to confer a risk of approximately 26%–35% (Miller 2002; Jones and Craddock 2001). Women with a history of both bipolar disorder and postpartum psychosis have a 38%–50% chance of recurrence of postpartum psychosis after subsequent deliveries (Jones and Craddock 2001; Rohde and Marneros 1992). A family history of postpartum psychosis and primiparity also increase the risk (Jones and Craddock 2001; O'Hara and Swain 1996), while a diagnosis of schizophrenia does not appear to be a significant risk factor (Miller 2002).

## Treatment

Because patients with postpartum psychosis are at risk for child neglect, child abuse, infanticide, and suicide, psychiatric hospitalization is almost always indicated. A medical assessment should be undertaken to rule out organic etiologies (e.g., postpartum thyroiditis, Sheehan's syndrome, intoxication/withdrawal states, pregnancy-related autoimmune disorders, an intracranial mass). Mood stabilizers should be initiated immediately, and antipsychotic agents are often necessary for acute psychosis and agitation. Although antidepressants are beneficial for patients with depressive psychosis, they should be used with caution in postpartum psychosis because there is a risk of precipitating a protracted and complicated course with rapid mood cycling (Sichel 1992). Electroconvulsive therapy is an important treatment alternative for patients who do not respond to pharmacotherapy or whose symptoms appear to be escalating.

Patients with a single episode of psychosis occurring in the postpartum period have a better long-term course than do patients with psychotic illnesses occurring at other times of their lives (Appleby et al. 1997). Nevertheless, the risk of subsequent mood episodes is relatively high. After an initial psychotic illness during the postpartum period, the probability of a recurrent affective illness has been reported to be approximately 60% (Davidson and Robertson 1985; Videbech and Gouliaev 1995). For a patient with a history of affective illness, maintenance treatment with a mood stabilizer is indicated. If there is no history of mood or psychotic episodes and if the patient prefers not to continue medication, mood stabilizers and/or antipsychotic agents can be tapered and discontinued at 9–12 months postpartum. The patient should be warned, however, of her risk of relapse and should be apprised as to the warning signs of recurrent illness. If she becomes pregnant again, mood stabilizers should be used prophylactically beginning at delivery if she is not already taking them. Although the proportion of first-episode postpartum psychoses that are eventually diagnosed as schizophrenia appears to be low (Videbech and Gouliaev 1995), women with schizophreniform symptoms in the postpartum period tend to have a serious mental illness (Davidson and Robertson 1985; Videbech and Gouliaev 1995) and may require maintenance treatment with an antipsychotic agent. Time of onset of symptoms influences the long-term prognosis: new-onset psychosis that develops within 3 weeks of delivery appears to have a more favorable course than a psychosis developing later in the postpartum period.

Patients with a history of bipolar disorder are at significant risk for postpartum psychosis. For these patients, initiation of a mood stabilizer either in the third trimester or immediately after delivery can significantly reduce the rate of relapse (Pfuhlmann et al. 2002). Researchers in a small study ($N=10$) reported success with estrogen administration for postpartum psychosis (Ahokas et al. 2000a), However, in a subsequent study ($N=29$), estrogen administration did not reduce the rate of relapse of postpartum psychosis (Kumar et al. 2003). At present the use of estrogen is not recommended for women with postpartum psychosis, particularly as it can reduce breast-milk volume and produce endometrial hyperplasia after only a few weeks of use.

# Etiology of Postpartum Mood Disorders

The etiology of postpartum mood disorders is unknown. A number of biological factors, including estrogen, progesterone, cortisol, tryptophan, thyroid hormones, β-endorphin, and prolactin, have been speculated to play a role, but studies have had negative or contradictory findings (Ahokas et al. 2000a; Ahokas et al. 2000b; Shear and Mammen 1995). In animal models, estrogen has an antidopaminergic effect, similar to that of antipsychotic agents (Gordon et al. 1980). An abrupt reduction of circulating estrogen levels, such as occurs after delivery, may produce dopamine receptor supersensitivity and thus predispose the patient to psychosis (Gordon et al. 1980).

Psychological factors probably play a role in postpartum depression. For example, the blues may reflect a letdown after the stress and excitement of pregnancy and childbirth (O'Hara 1995). Psychological factors that may increase vulnerability to postpartum depressive symptoms include a low sense of self-control and maladaptive cognitions (O'Hara 1995). Although incidence rates of postpartum psychosis appear consistent across cultures and ethnic groups (Ahokas et al. 2000b), postpartum depression is reported to occur less frequently in some non-Western societies. In particular, rates of postpartum depression appear lower in cultures where women receive assistance, appreciation of their new roles as mothers, education about the techniques of mothering, and an opportunity to rest after the delivery (Kruckman 1992). It is unlikely that a single etiology accounts for postpartum mood disorders. Biological, social, and psychological factors probably contribute—to varying degrees in different women.

## Postpartum Anxiety Disorders

Postpartum anxiety disorders have been studied less extensively than mood disorders, and no data exist at present on their prevalence. However, a number of case reports have described new onset or exacerbation of anxiety disorders, in particular panic disorder and obsessive-compulsive disorder (Shear and Mammen 1995). The onset or worsening of symptoms typically occurs in the first 12 weeks after delivery. A common theme underlying obsessions occurring during the postpartum is fear of harming the child. These obsessions produce significant distress, and women may be ashamed to reveal them. In contrast to postpartum psychosis, which may also involve thoughts of harming the baby, the obsessions of postpartum obsessive-compulsive disorder cause significant distress to the mother but pose no risk to the child.

As for postpartum depression, the treatment of postpartum anxiety disorders should be multifactorial. Cognitive-behavioral therapy and interpersonal therapy can be very helpful and may preclude the need for medications. For women who require pharmacological treatment, the agents that are routinely used for anxiety disorders (e.g., serotonergic antidepressants, tricyclic antidepressants, benzodiazepines, buspirone) are effective for postpartum anxiety disorders. Treatment should be continued for a minimum of 9–12 months after remission of symptoms. More research remains to be done on the long-term course of these disorders.

## Breast-Feeding and Psychotropic Medications

About 50% of new mothers breast-feed. Breast-feeding not only enhances maternal-infant bonding but also offers health benefits to the baby. Breast milk contains antibodies, enzymes, hormones, growth factors, and other compounds that foster maturation of the infant's digestive tract (Goldman 1993) and protect against pathogens. Respiratory and urinary tract infections occur less frequently in breast-fed infants than in those who are bottle-fed. However, because little is known about the risks to an infant of exposure to medications through breast milk, clinicians and patients often choose to forgo breast-feeding. Fortunately, data on the use of psychotropic medication in breast-feeding women are increasingly reassuring, because more case reports note no adverse effects in lactating infants exposed to medication. Nevertheless, no medication should be used by a breast-feeding woman without a careful consideration of the risks and benefits.

Other treatment approaches, including individual and group psychotherapy and reduction of psychosocial stressors, should be attempted before psychotropic agents are used. If these approaches fail, or if the woman chooses to use medication after being thoroughly informed of alternative treatments, a careful discussion with the woman and her partner should ensue. This discussion should review the available data on breast-feeding and psychotropic medication use, including what is known about risks and benefits. It is important that a pediatrician who is aware of the breast-feeding mother's use of medication monitor the infant for potential adverse sequelae.

To establish the infant's baseline of behavior, sleep and feeding patterns, and alertness, a pediatric assessment should be obtained before breast-feeding is begun. Infant drug clearance increases from approximately 33% of the mother's weight-adjusted clearance at birth to 100% at about age 6 months. Therefore, treatment of the nursing mother of a neonate may be riskier than that of a woman whose baby is older. In general, it is prudent for the mother of a premature infant *not* to nurse if she is taking psychotropic medications, because the infant's liver enzyme production is likely to be immature. To minimize the infant's exposure to medication, the mother should be prescribed the minimum dose of medication that achieves remission of her psychiatric symptoms. If her symptoms do not improve with pharmacotherapy, a reevaluation of the risk-benefit discussion is warranted.

Other considerations in the use of psychotropic medications while breast-feeding include the use of short-acting rather than long-acting medications, use of medications without active metabolites, and supplementation with bottle-feeding to reduce the infant's exposure to the drug.

Studies evaluating serum concentrations of antidepressants in nursing infants have typically found low concentrations, particularly for sertraline, paroxetine, and citalopram (Berle et al. 2004). Therefore, routine monitoring of serum concentrations does not appear necessary for nursing infants whose mothers take these agents. However, serum concentrations can be measured if the mother feels that the data will bring reassurance. To obtain an infant's serum concentration of medication, the procedure is as follows: Once the mother's medication serum level is at steady state, the infant's serum should be assayed for *concentrations* of both the parent drug and its metabolites. Laboratories should be requested to use high-sensitivity assays (preferably with limits of detection <2 ng/mL). At present, no cutoff level has been established for concern about serum concentrations of antidepressant medications in infants. In the absence of adverse effects in the infant, there appears to be no reason for a woman to discontinue nursing regardless of the infant's serum concentration.

Table 5–4 summarizes current knowledge on the use of psychotropic medications by breast-feeding women. Most psychiatric medications have been classified by the American Academy of Pediatrics (AAP) as "drugs whose effect on nursing infants is unknown but may be of concern" (American Academy of Pediatrics Committee on Drugs 2001). These medications include the tricyclic antidepressants, benzodiazepines, and antipsychotic agents.

**Table 5–4.**    Psychotropic drugs taken during breast-feeding

| Medication | Comment | References |
|---|---|---|
| **Antidepressants** | | |
| Tricyclic antidepressants | In most cases, parent compound levels in infant serum are below limits of detection, but metabolite levels are sometimes detectable. One case of respiratory depression was noted in an infant exposed to doxepin through breast milk. | Burt et al. 2001; Matheson et al. 1985; Misri and Kostaras 2002 |
| Selective serotonin reuptake inhibitors | Data for fluoxetine consist of more than 190 exposures, including 10 reports of adverse events per maternal report. In 9 of these cases, the infants experienced colic-like symptoms. No adverse effects were noted with sertraline (90+ infants), paroxetine (100+ infants), fluvoxamine (seven infants), citalopram (51 infants). | Aichhorn et al. 2004; Berle et al. 2004; Burt et al. 2001; Hendrick et al. 2001a; Hendrick et al. 2001b; Kristensen et al. 1999; Lee et al. 2004; Lester et al. 1993; Stowe et al. 2000; Stowe et al. 2003 |
| Other antidepressants | No adverse effects noted with bupropion (3 infants, a possible seizure in a 6-month-old infant), venlafaxine (12 infants), nefazodone (1 infant), and mirtazapine (1 infant). No published data for duloxetine. | Burt et al. 2001; Baab et al. 2002; Chaudron and Schoenecker 2004; Ilett et al. 2002; Yapp et al. 2000 |
| St. John's wort | Two case reports with no adverse effects. | Klier et al. 2002; Lee et al. 2003 |

**Table 5–4.** Psychotropic drugs taken during breast-feeding *(continued)*

| Medication | Comment | References |
|---|---|---|
| **Antianxiety agents** | | |
| Benzodiazepines | Benzodiazepines (especially long-acting agents) may accumulate in neonates because of their immature liver enzymes. Occasional low doses of short-acting benzodiazepines (e.g., lorazepam, oxazepam, temazepam) are unlikely to be harmful. Reports of sedation and lethargy have been noted with diazepam (2 infants), and irritability and possible withdrawal have been noted with alprazolam (1 infant). Cyanosis and impaired respiration (reversible) have been noted with clonazepam (1 infant). | Burt at al. 2001; McElhatton et al. 1994 |
| Zolpidem | In five cases of exposure through breast milk, no adverse effects were noted. More data are needed before recommendations can be made for this agent. | Burt et al. 2001 |
| Gabapentin | No data are available. | |

**Table 5–4.    Psychotropic drugs taken during breast-feeding (continued)**

| Medication | Comment | References |
|---|---|---|
| Antipsychotic agents | No adverse effects were observed in 42 infants exposed to olanzapine through breast milk. The median dose of olanzapine in breast milk to which infants were exposed was 1.02% of the maternal dose. None of the infants had a detectable level of olanzapine in the blood sample. Lethargy developed in 1 infant exposed to chlorpromazine; developmental delay between 12 and 18 months was noted in 3 infants exposed to high doses of haloperidol plus chlorpromazine. Clozapine accumulated in breast milk of 1 mother exposed to this agent (no notation of effect on infant). The American Academy of Pediatrics (AAP) considers chlorpromazine, haloperidol, and mesoridazine to be in the category of drugs whose effect on nursing infants is unknown but may be of concern. The AAP has not published recommendations regarding the other antipsychotic agents. No adverse effects in two cases of risperidone use. No data are available on use of ziprasidone and aripiprazole. | Barnas et al. 1994; Buist 2001; Burt et al. 2001; Gardiner et al. 2003; Gentile 2004; Goldstein et al. 2000; Hill et al. 2000; Ilett et al. 2004; Ratnayake and Libretto 2002; Yoshida et al. 1998 |

**Table 5–4.** Psychotropic drugs taken during breast-feeding (*continued*)

| Medication | Comment | References |
|---|---|---|
| **Mood stabilizers** | | |
| Lithium | Concentration in milk may reach up to 77% of the concentration in maternal plasma. Because neonatal kidney is immature, risk for lithium accumulation is high. One infant with a congenital heart murmur who was exposed to lithium both in utero and through breast milk exhibited electrocardiogram changes, which resolved after lithium was discontinued. The AAP considers lithium contraindicated during breast-feeding. | Burt et al. 2001; Buist 2001; Dodd and Berk 2004; Gentile 2004 |
| Carbamazepine | Rapidly metabolized, does not appear in infant serum. The AAP considers this drug compatible with breast-feeding. Nevertheless, transient hepatic dysfunction has been noted in two infants exposed to carbamazepine. Carbamazepine use by breast-feeding mothers therefore requires careful clinical and laboratory monitoring of nurslings. | Burt et al. 2001; Frey et al. 2002; Merlob et al. 1992 |

**Table 5–4.**    Psychotropic drugs taken during breast-feeding *(continued)*

| Medication | Comment | References |
|---|---|---|
| Valproate | The AAP considers this drug compatible with breast-feeding. However, thrombocytopenia and anemia in a 3-month-old infant breast-fed by a mother taking this agent reversed after nursing was discontinued. Concerns of toxicity in infants suggest caution and careful clinical and laboratory monitoring (liver enzymes, complete blood count, platelets) when breast-feeding women are administered this agent. | Burt et al. 2001; Dodd and Berk 2004 |
| Lamotrigine | No adverse effects have been noted, but blood levels in infants can reach adult levels, possibly because of infants' inefficient glucuronidation. | Burt et al. 2001; Liporace et al. 2004; Ohman et al. 2000 |
| Topiramate | In five cases, no adverse effects were noted. | Ohman et al. 2002 |

Since postpartum depression is fairly common, it is reassuring that accumulating data show that the use of antidepressants by breast-feeding mothers is relatively safe. Medications for which extensive safety data exist (e.g., paroxetine, sertraline, citalopram) should be used as first-line agents for breast-feeding women requiring antidepressants. Although monoamine oxidase inhibitors are not included in the AAP's listing, they should not be used during breast-feeding because of the risk of hypertension in the infant. A recent case report described successful treatment of major depression during pregnancy with omega-3 polyunsaturated fatty acids (4 g/day of ethyl eicosapentaenoic acid and 2 g/day of docosahexaenoic acid) (Chiu et al. 2003). Omega-3 polyunsaturated fatty acids offer significant health benefits to nursing women and their infants. An adequate supply of maternal docosahexaenoic acid during nursing is necessary to support the optimal neurological development of the infant. If the preliminary data on omega-3 fatty acids' positive mood effects are corroborated in larger studies, they may become a safe and healthful treatment option for depression in pregnant and nursing women.

Bipolar disorder is best treated with mood stabilizers. However, the use of mood stabilizers in postpartum nursing women is problematic because these medications have been associated with serious sequelae in nursing babies. The AAP lists carbamazepine and sodium valproate among drugs that "are usually compatible with breast-feeding" (American Academy of Pediatrics Committee on Drugs 2001). However, exposure to valproate has been associated with hepatotoxicity in infants and also with one case of thrombocytopenia and anemia, and carbamazepine has been reported to be associated with hepatic dysfunction. Therefore, breast-feeding women should use these agents with caution, and nurslings should be monitored clinically and with liver function checks for possible liver toxicity. The AAP lists lithium as contraindicated during nursing because adverse effects—including cardiotoxicity, dehydration, and lithium toxicity—have been noted in infants exposed to lithium.

Postpartum psychosis should be treated with antipsychotic agents and often requires additional psychotropic medications. Women who require antipsychotic agents during the postpartum period tend to be severely ill. Since breast-feeding requires the intensive attention of the mother and is associated with significant sleep deprivation, postpartum women who are taking antipsychotic medications should generally be encouraged not to breast-feed their infants.

# References

Ahokas A, Aito M, Rimon R: Positive treatment effect of estradiol in postpartum psychosis: a pilot study. J Clin Psychiatry 61:166–169, 2000a

Ahokas A, Aito M, Turiainen S: Association between oestradiol and puerperal psychosis. Acta Psychiatr Scand 101:167–169, 2000b

Ahokas A, Kaukoranta J, Wahlbeck K, et al: Estrogen deficiency in severe postpartum depression: successful treatment with sublingual physiologic 17beta-estradiol: a preliminary study. J Clin Psychiatry 62:332–336, 2001

Aichhorn W, Whitworth AB, Weiss U, et al: Mirtazapine and breast-feeding (letter). Am J Psychiatry 161:2325, 2004

American Academy of Pediatrics Committee on Drugs: The transfer of drugs and other chemicals into human milk. Pediatrics 108:776–789, 2001

Appleby L, Warner R, Whitton A, et al: A controlled study of fluoxetine and cognitive-behavioural counselling in the treatment of postnatal depression. BMJ 314:932–936, 1997

Baab SW, Peindl KS, Piontek CM, et al: Serum bupropion levels in 2 breastfeeding mother-infant pairs. J Clin Psychiatry 63:910–911, 2002

Barnas C, Bergant A, Hummer M, et al: Clozapine concentrations in maternal and fetal plasma, amniotic fluid, and breast milk (letter). Am J Psychiatry 151:945, 1994

Berle JO, Steen VM, Aamo TO, et al: Breastfeeding during maternal antidepressant treatment with serotonin reuptake inhibitors: infant exposure, clinical symptoms, and cytochrome p450 genotypes. J Clin Psychiatry 65:1228–1234, 2004

Brennan PA, Hammen C, Andersen MJ, et al: Chronicity, severity, and timing of maternal depressive symptoms: relationships with child outcomes at age 5. Dev Psychol 36:759–766, 2000

Buist A: Treating mental illness in lactating women. Medscape Womens Health 6:3, 2001

Burt VK, Suri R, Altshuler L, et al: The use of psychotropic medications during breast-feeding. Am J Psychiatry 158:1001–1009, 2001

Chaudron LH, Pies RW: The relationship between postpartum psychosis and bipolar disorder: a review. J Clin Psychiatry 64:1284–1292, 2003

Chaudron LH, Schoenecker CJ: Bupropion and breastfeeding: a case of a possible infant seizure (letter). J Clin Psychiatry 65:881–882, 2004

Chiu CC, Huang SY, Shen WW, et al: Omega-3 fatty acids for depression in pregnancy (letter). Am J Psychiatry 160:385, 2003

Cohen LS, Viguera AC, Bouffard SM, et al: Venlafaxine in the treatment of postpartum depression. J Clin Psychiatry 62:592–596, 2001

Cooper P, Murray L: Prediction, detection, and treatment of postnatal depression. Arch Dis Child 77:97–99, 1997

Corral M, Kuan A, Kostaras D: Bright light therapy's effect on postpartum depression (letter). Am J Psychiatry 157:303–304, 2000

Davidson J, Robertson E: A follow-up study of postpartum illness, 1946–1978. Acta Psychiatr Scand 71:451–457, 1985

Dodd S, Berk M: The pharmacology of bipolar disorder during pregnancy and breast-feeding. Expert Opin Drug Saf 3:221–229, 2004

Field T, Lang C, Martinez A, et al: Preschool follow-up of children of dysphoric mothers. J Clin Child Psychol 25:275–279, 1996

Field T, Pickens J, Prodromidis M, et al: Targeting adolescent mothers with depressive symptoms for early intervention. Adolescence 35:381–414, 2000

Frey B, Braegger CP, Ghelfi D: Neonatal cholestatic hepatitis from carbamazepine exposure during pregnancy and breast feeding. Ann Pharmacother 36:644–647, 2002

Gardiner SJ, Kristensen JH, Begg EJ, et al: Transfer of olanzapine into breast milk, calculation of infant drug dose, and effect on breast-fed infants. Am J Psychiatry 160:1428–1431, 2003

Gentile S: Clinical utilization of atypical antipsychotics in pregnancy and lactation. Ann Pharmacother 38:1265–1271, 2004

Goldman AS: The immune system of human milk: antimicrobial, antiinflammatory and immunomodulating properties. Pediatr Infect Dis J 12:664–671, 1993

Goldstein DJ, Corbin LA, Fung MC: Olanzapine-exposed pregnancies and lactation: early experience. J Clin Psychopharmacol 20:399–403, 2000

Gordon JH, Borison RL, Diamond B: Modulation of dopamine receptor sensitivity by estrogen. Biol Psychiatry 15:389–396, 1980

Grace, SL, Evindar A, Stewart DE: The effect of postpartum depression on child cognitive development and behavior: a review and critical analysis of the literature. Arch Womens Ment Health 6:263–274, 2003

Gregoire AJ, Kumar R, Everitt B, et al: Transdermal oestrogen for treatment of severe postnatal depression. Lancet 347:930–933, 1996

Hendrick V, Stowe ZN, Altshuler LL, et al: Fluoxetine and norfluoxetine concentrations in nursing infants and breast milk. Biol Psychiatry 50:775–782, 2001a

Hendrick V, Fukuchi A, Altshuler LL, et al: Use of sertraline, paroxetine and fluvoxamine by nursing women. Br J Psychiatry 179: 163–166, 2001b

Hendrick V, Smith LM, Hwang S, et al: Weight gain in breastfed infants of mothers taking antidepressant medications. J Clin Psychiatry 64:410–412, 2003

Hill RC, McIvor RJ, Wojnar-Horton RE, et al: Risperidone distribution and excretion into human milk: case report and estimated infant exposure during breast-feeding. J Clin Psychopharmacol 20:285–286, 2000

Ilett KF, Kristensen JH, Hackett LP, et al: Distribution of venlafaxine and its O-desmethyl metabolite in human milk and their effects in breastfed infants. Br J Clin Pharmacol 53:17–22, 2002

Ilett KF, Hackett LP, Kristensen JH, et al: Transfer of risperidone and 9-hydroxyrisperidone into human milk. Ann Pharmacother 38:273–276, 2004

Jones I, Craddock N: Familiarity of the puerperal trigger in bipolar disorder: results of a family study. Am J Psychiatry 158:913–917, 2001

Klier CM, Schafer MR, Schmid-Siegel B, et al: St. John's wort (*Hypericum perforatum*)—is it safe during breastfeeding? Pharmacopsychiatry 35:29–30, 2002

Kristensen JH, Ilett KI, Hackett LP, et al: Distribution and excretion of fluoxetine and norfluoxetine in human milk. Br J Clin Pharmacol 48:521–527, 1999

Kruckman LD: Rituals and support: an anthropological view of postpartum depression, in Postpartum Psychiatric Illness: A Picture Puzzle. Edited by Hamilton JA, Harberger PN. Philadelphia, PA, University of Pennsylvania Press, 1992, pp 137–148

Kumar C, McIvor RJ, Davies T, et al: Estrogen administration does not reduce the rate of recurrence of affective psychosis after childbirth. J Clin Psychiatry 64:112–118, 2003

Lawrie TA, Herxheimer A, Dalton K: Oestrogens and progestogens for preventing and treating postnatal depression. Cochrane Database Syst Rev 2:CD001690, 2000

Lee A, Minhas R, Noriko M, et al: The safety of St. John's wort (*Hypericum perforatum*) during breastfeeding. J Clin Psychiatry 64:966–968, 2003

Lee A, Woo J, Ito S: Frequency of infant adverse events that are associated with citalopram use during breast-feeding. Am J Obstet Gynecol 190:218–221, 2004

Lester BM, Cucca J, Andreozzi BA, et al: Possible association between fluoxetine hydrochloride and colic in an infant. J Am Acad Child Adolesc Psychiatry 32:1253–1255, 1993

Liporace J, Kao A, D'breu A: Concerns regarding lamotrigine and breast-feeding. Epilepsy Behav 5:102–105, 2004

Lyons-Ruth K, Wolfe R, Lyubchik A, et al: Depressive symptoms in parents of children under age three: sociodemographic predictors, current correlates and associated parenting behaviors. in Child-Rearing in America: Challenges Facing Parents With Young Children. Edited by Halfon N, Schuster M, Taaffe Young K. New York, Cambridge University Press, 2002, pp 217–262

Matheson I, Pande H, Alertsen AR: Respiratory depression caused by N-desmethyldoxepin in breast milk (letter). Lancet 2:1124, 1985

McElhatton PR: The effects of benzodiazepine use during pregnancy and lactation. Reprod Toxicol 8:461–475, 1994

Merlob P, Mor M, Litwin A: Transient hepatic dysfunction in an infant of an epileptic mother treated with carbamazepine during pregnancy and breastfeeding. Ann Pharmacother 26:1563–1565, 1992

Miller LJ: Postpartum depression. JAMA 287:762–765, 2002

Misri S, Kostaras X: Benefits and risks to mother and infant of drug treatment for postnatal depression. Drug Saf 25:903–911, 2002

O'Hara MW: Postpartum Depression: Causes and Consequences. New York, Springer-Verlag, 1995

O'Hara MW, Swain AM: Rates and risk of postpartum depression—a meta-analysis. International Review of Psychiatry 8: 37–54, 1996

O'Hara MW, Stuart S, Gorman LL, et al: Efficacy of interpersonal psychotherapy for postpartum depression. Arch Gen Psychiatry 57:1039–1045, 2000

Ohman I, Vitols S, Tomson T: Lamotrigine in pregnancy: pharmacokinetics during delivery, in the neonate, and during lactation. Epilepsia 41:709–713, 2000

Ohman I, Vitols S, Luef G, et al: Topiramate kinetics during delivery, lactation, and in the neonate: preliminary observations. Epilepsia 43:1157–1160, 2002

Pfuhlmann B, Stoeber G, Beckmann H: Postpartum psychoses: prognosis, risk factors, and treatment. Curr Psychiatry Rep 4:185–190, 2002

Ratnayake T, Libretto SE: No complications with risperidone treatment before and throughout pregnancy and during the nursing period (letter). J Clin Psychiatry 63:76–77, 2002

Rohde A, Marneros A: Schizoaffective disorders with and without onset in the puerperium. Eur Arch Psychiatry Clin Neurosci 242:27–33, 1992

Rupprecht R, Holsboer F: Neuropsychopharmacological properties of neuroactive steroids. Steroids 64:83–91, 1999

Segre LS, Stuart S, O'Hara MW: Interpersonal psychotherapy for antenatal and postpartum depression. Primary Psychiatry 11:52–56, 66, 2004

Shear MK, Mammen O: Anxiety disorders in pregnant and postpartum women. Psychopharmacol Bull 31:693–703, 1995

Sichel DA: Psychiatric issues in the postpartum period. Currents in Affective Illness 11:5–12, 1992

Sinclair D, Murray L: Effects of postnatal depression on children's adjustment to school: teacher's reports. Br J Psychiatry 172:58–63, 1998

Stagnaro-Green A: Postpartum thryoiditis. J Clin Endocrin Metab 87:4042–4047, 2002

Stowe ZN, Cohen LS, Hostetter A, et al: Paroxetine in human breast milk and nursing infants. Am J Psychiatry 157:185–189, 2000

Stowe ZN, Hostetter AL, Owens MJ, et al: The pharmacokinetics of sertraline excretion into human breast milk: determinants of infant serum concentrations. J Clin Psychiatry 64:73–80, 2003

Videbech P, Gouliaev G: First admission with puerperal psychosis: 7–14 years of follow-up. Acta Psychiatr Scand 91:167–173, 1995

Wisner KL, Wheeler SB: Prevention of recurrent postpartum major depression. Hosp Community Psychiatry 45:1191–1196, 1994

Wisner KL, Perel JM, Peindl KS, et al: Prevention of recurrent postpartum depression: a randomized clinical trial. J Clin Psychiatry 62: 82–86, 2001

Yapp P, Ilett KF, Kristensen JH, et al: Drowsiness and poor feeding in a breast-fed infant: association with nefazodone and its metabolites. Ann Pharmacother 34:1269–1272, 2000

Yoshida K, Smith B, Craggs M, et al: Neuroleptic drugs in breast-milk: a study of pharmacokinetics and of possible adverse effects in breast-fed infants. Psychol Med 28:81–91, 1998

Zelkowitz P, Milet TH: The course of postpartum psychiatric disorders in women and their partners. J Nerv Ment Dis 189:575–582, 2001

# 6

# Induced Abortion and Pregnancy Loss

## Induced Abortion

Induced abortion is the deliberate termination of pregnancy. The landmark U.S. Supreme Court decision *Roe v. Wade* (1973) allowed women to terminate pregnancy in the first trimester, after which individual state laws prevail. Before and since that time, controversy has raged across the United States regarding a woman's right to choose abortion. Approximately one of five women in the United States has had a legal abortion (Major et al. 2000).

### Epidemiology

In the United States, most women who elect to have an abortion are single and under age 25 years (Strauss et al. 2004).

Since 1984, 11 years following the legalization of induced abortion, the percentage of pregnancies ending in abortion has dropped steadily. In 2001, the Centers for Disease Control and Prevention recorded 246 induced abortions per 1,000 live births. This decline in the abortion ratio may be explained by attitudinal changes toward elective abortion; more available, acceptable, and effective contraceptive methods (including emergency contraception performed the day after unprotected sex); reduced access to abortion services; and a decline in unplanned pregnancies (Strauss et al. 2004).

In 1999, a total of 88% of elective abortions were performed within the first trimester of pregnancy, and 98% were performed before the 21st week

(Grimes and Creinin 2004). Data for 2001 from the Centers for Disease Control and Prevention revealed that 59% of abortions were performed at or before 8 weeks' gestation and that 1.4% occurred after 21 weeks' gestation (Strauss et al. 2004). A 1987 survey of abortion patients across the United States found that one-half of the survey respondents were practicing contraception during the month in which they conceived (Henshaw and Silverman 1988). The patients who did not use contraception were more likely to be young, poor, black, or Hispanic and were less educated than users of contraception.

## Abortion Techniques, Mortality, and Morbidity

The method used for the vast majority of abortions involves either the administration of a medication prescribed by a health professional ("medical abortion") or dilatation of the cervix and evacuation of the uterine contents by means of vacuum aspiration or curettage ("surgical abortion") (Stotland 2001). First-trimester abortions and most second-trimester abortions are accomplished by vacuum aspiration under local anesthesia in free-standing clinics (Grimes and Creinin 2004).

Medical abortions are most effective within the first 7 weeks of pregnancy. Termination of the pregnancy occurs by precipitation of uterine contractions and thus emptying the uterus of the products of conception. One medical method for termination of early pregnancy includes the use of the agent mifepristone (RU486), which causes the placenta to separate from the uterine lining (endometrium) by competing with progesterone for uterine receptor sites. In September 2000, the U.S. Food and Drug Administration (FDA) approved the use of mifepristone for termination of pregnancies of less than 49 days' gestation. The FDA further stipulated that 2 days after mifepristone administration, patients must return for a dose of the prostaglandin E analogue misoprostol. Other agents, which are currently available for indications other than abortion, have been used off-label to induce early abortions. These agents include the folic acid analogue methotrexate, which is given in conjunction with misoprostol. A follow-up examination is generally done 2–3 weeks after a medical abortion and often includes a physical examination to check both the cervix and the uterus, an evaluation of the blood level of β-human chorionic gonadotropin (β-HCG) to confirm that the pregnancy has ended, a blood test to check for anemia, and a discussion of birth control. If the patient desires, an intrauterine device may be inserted at this time. Although both mifepristone and methotrexate are effective inducers of abortion, mifepristone has fewer side effects. Medical abortions have a success rate of greater than 90%. If a medical abortion fails or some products of conception are retained in the uterus, surgery must be done to prevent complications. It is likely that in the near future many more abortions will be performed medically (Westfall 1998).

Surgical abortion generally involves suction (vacuum) aspiration of the contents of the uterus. Suction is accomplished either manually or with the assistance of a vacuum apparatus designed to provide gentle vacuum. Dilatation and curettage (D and C) is done to remove tissue from inside the uterus during the first 12 weeks of pregnancy; it is the least common type of surgical abortion done during the first trimester. This procedure is also used to remove tissue remaining in the uterus after a miscarriage or to remove tissue within the uterus that may be causing abnormal uterine bleeding. The D and C procedure involves the administration of anesthesia, dilation of the cervix, passing of a curved instrument (curette) into the uterus, and gentle scraping the uterine lining. Antibiotics are usually given after a D and C to prevent infection. Suction aspiration is more commonly used in the first trimester because it is safer than a D and C. Occasionally a D and C may be done after suction aspiration if not all tissue has been removed.

The mortality rate from elective abortion is approximately 0.4 per 100,000 procedures and is less risky than carrying a pregnancy to term. It is noteworthy that the rate of mortality from childbirth is 25 times greater than that from elective abortion. Risk factors for complications include older maternal age, non-Caucasian race, older gestational age, and techniques of abortion other than aspiration or curettage. Although the years since 1940 have been characterized by a decline in deaths caused by complications from childbirth and abortion, the abortion mortality ratio for women (abortions per 1,000 live births) has declined more rapidly than has the rate of mortality from childbirth. The steepest drop in women's mortality resulting from abortion occurred since 1967–1970, the years corresponding to the liberalization of state abortion laws (Frank et al. 1987).

Induced abortion is not associated with an increased risk of subsequent infertility. In addition, prior elective abortion has no effect on the rate of subsequent pregnancy-related morbidity, including spontaneous abortion, premature delivery, and low-birth-weight infants (Grimes and Creinin 2004).

## Reasons for Induced Abortion

Women elect to have an abortion for a number of reasons, including an inability to support a child financially, lack of willingness or ability to assume the responsibility for a child, lack of social supports, impregnation by incest or rape, reluctance to be a single parent, conflicts with a partner, and diagnosis of a fetal congenital anomaly.

## Prenatal Diagnosis and Induced Abortion

Prenatal diagnostic tests are used for a variety of reasons, including dating of the pregnancy, assessment of fetal anomalies, location of the placenta, and determination of amniotic fluid volume. Maternal serum screening performed between the seventh and fourteenth week of pregnancy reveals risks for a number of fetal malformations and Down syndrome. The ultrasound marker, nuchal translucency, measured in weeks 10–14 has been shown (together with maternal age) to detect 83.3% of Down syndrome fetuses with a false positive rate of 8.3%. Furthermore, in combination with several maternal serum markers, ultrasonographic calculation of fetal nuchal thickness increases the detection rate for Down syndrome to more than 90% with a false positive rate of 5% (Christiansen et al. 2004). When prenatal tests reveal serious congenital anomalies, consideration is usually given to termination of the pregnancy. If a decision is made to continue with the pregnancy, knowledge before the delivery allows time to adjust to a difficult outcome. Indications and timing for prenatal diagnostic tests are summarized in Table 6–1.

## Psychological Effects of Elective Abortion

An undesired pregnancy is a major crisis in a woman's life, and this crisis is often resolved by termination of the pregnancy. Structured tests to evaluate mood and well-being in women have shown improved scores immediately after abortion and for years thereafter (Dagg 1991; Westhoff et al. 2003).

Although most women experience few or no adverse psychological sequelae after an elective abortion, some women do experience postabortion psychological distress. For women who have undergone an elective first-

**Table 6–1.** Prenatal diagnostic tests

| | Indications | Timing | Risk of Fetal Loss |
|---|---|---|---|
| Maternal serum analyte screening: assays for maternal serum α-fetoprotein, β-human chorionic gonadotropin (β-HCG) unconjugated estriol (uE$_3$), inhibin A, pregnancy-associated protein A (PAPP-A) | All patients: to screen for incorrect dating, multiple gestation, neural tube defects, certain fetal chromosomal abnormalities (e.g., trisomy 21, trisomy 18), other fetal anomalies, fetal death | 15–20 weeks of gestation | 0 |
| Fetal ultrasound (fetal nuchal translucency and other sonographic–detectable physical markers) | Level I (basic) ultrasound: uncertain gestational age, location and grade of placenta, number of fetuses, cardiac activity, amniotic fluid volume, vaginal bleeding, detection of gross fetal abnormalities | Varies: early in first trimester or any other time | 0 |
| | Level II (targeted) ultrasound: previous fetus or infant with congenital anomaly, family history of congenital anomaly, in utero exposure to any potential teratogen (e.g., valproic acid, carbamazepine, lithium) | 18–20 weeks of gestation | 0 |

**Table 6–1.** Prenatal diagnostic tests *(continued)*

| | Indications | Timing | Risk of Fetal Loss |
|---|---|---|---|
| Amniocentesis | Maternal age at least 35 years, abnormal maternal serum analyte screening, history of chromosomal anomaly in fetus or infant, chromosomal abnormality in parent, family history of detectable Mendelian disorder | 12–20 weeks of gestation | 1–2 (12–15 weeks of gestation) 0.5–1.0 (15–20 weeks of gestation) |
| Chorionic villus sampling | Maternal age at least 35 years, history of chromosomal anomaly in previous fetus or infant, chromosomal abnormality in parent, family history of detectable Mendelian disorder, history of three or more spontaneous abortions | 9–13 weeks of gestation | 0.5–1.5 |

trimester abortion, the strongest predictor of poor postabortion psychological outcome is a prepregnancy history of depression (Major et al. 2000). Other factors increasing the likelihood of negative emotional experiences include medical or genetic indications for the abortion, an abortion performed at mid-trimester (especially if induction of labor and delivery were required for termination of the pregnancy), ambivalence about the decision to abort, and a feeling that the decision was not freely made (Dagg 1991). Although there have been reports of a "postabortion syndrome" analogous to posttraumatic stress disorder (PTSD) (Speckhard and Rue 1992), most studies suggest that freely chosen abortion, especially in the first trimester, does not result in postabortion psychopathology. Data from a comprehensive 2-year prospective study of first-trimester postabortion responses indicated that the rate of PTSD in the subjects was lower than the rate in a general age-matched female population (Major et al. 2000).

## Abortion Counseling

### The Purpose of Abortion Counseling

Having an abortion is a momentous event for most women, and abortion counseling is an important component of the abortion procedure. Counseling sessions provide an opportunity to assess available options, screen for psychological difficulties or serious psychopathology, offer information regarding the abortion procedure, and review ways to prevent future unplanned pregnancies. Counseling also gives women an opportunity to express and assimilate feelings connected with the relationship in which pregnancy occurred and issues connected with abortion as a possible outcome. For women who choose abortion, counseling minimizes preoperative anxiety and hastens postoperative recovery.

Many women who consider abortion have questions about the procedure and mixed feelings about their choice. It is important that the setting for abortion be both medically safe and psychologically supportive. It is common and understandable for women to have concerns about the safety of abortion, the extent of pain and discomfort present during or after the procedure, and possible sequelae. In this regard, abortion counseling—besides offering psychological support—provides information about the procedure itself and about possible complications. For this reason, the abortion counselor should understand reproductive physiology and be knowledgeable about abortion procedures. A primary care practitioner may help a woman decide what procedure (medical or surgical) she prefers and prepare her for what to expect (Stotland 2002).

For the most part, patients in their first trimester of pregnancy tend to experience less stress than do those in the second trimester. Individuals in the latter group are more likely to be young, poor, and unfamiliar with gynecological procedures (Hern 1990). All patients should be given the opportunity to discuss their reasons for considering an abortion. For patients who are ambivalent or who present for abortion to satisfy parents or a partner but who have not truly explored what they want for themselves, it is essential to provide an open opportunity for discussion of the alternatives available to pregnant women.

Although most women who have abortions do not experience negative psychological sequelae, some experience a heightened awareness of interpersonal or other difficulties in their lives. Many women who decide to proceed with abortion do not want and do not require further counseling after the abortion. Nevertheless, it is useful at least to offer options for ongoing counseling should the patient request further assistance.

### The Process of Abortion Counseling

The patient who presents for abortion counseling should be encouraged to examine her feelings concerning the pregnancy, the prospect of abortion, the relationship in which the pregnancy occurred, and possible feelings after the abortion has been completed. The basic anatomy and physiology of reproduction should be reviewed, and the abortion procedure itself should be discussed. The patient should be aware of how to obtain both medical and psychological follow-up assistance, should these be needed. Options for subsequent birth control should be carefully discussed, and the risks and benefits of each alternative reviewed.

Women whose pregnancy resulted from rape are likely to experience psychological difficulties because they are pregnant and also because they have been raped. Although abortion counseling is an appropriate and necessary part of the mental health process, these patients often require additional mental health care to address psychological sequelae of their traumatic experience. As with all women who present for abortion, feelings should be explored. Information about the procedure and its risks and possible complications should be reviewed. Provision should be made for follow-up rape crisis counseling.

Another difficult situation that occurs in the setting of abortion counseling is that of the woman who requests an abortion because of a severe fetal deformity or impending fetal death. Such women should be given ample opportunity to express their feelings. After the decision to abort an abnormal fetus, women may experience mourning for the loss of a wished-for baby, and they often benefit from bereavement counseling. In some cases, guilt for having produced a deformed fetus may require sensitive exploration and resolution (Zolese and Blacker 1992). Decision making about subsequent pregnancies may be fraught with ambivalence, fear, and anxiety, and women may need close follow-up with mental health professionals over the course of future pregnancies. The clinician must be patient and empathic. Communication between the mental health counselor and the obstetrician is essential so that the woman can be given reassurance and support by clinicians who fully understand the obstetrical complications encountered by the patient. Also included in the therapy should be the woman's partner, who may also be grieving but who may come to be relied on as a source of support for the pregnant partner rather than being treated as a person in need of psychological support. Providing abortion counseling requires a team effort. Ideally, the team includes the patient, her partner, the gynecologist, and a skilled and sensitive mental health counselor with knowledge of reproductive physiology and abortion procedures.

The pregnant woman with a severe and chronic mental illness presents special issues for the abortion counselor. Such patients should be assessed by a psychiatrist with experience in addressing issues concerning pregnancy in women with psychotic disorders. Evaluation should address ongoing delusions, paranoia, and hallucinations. The ability of the patient to understand her pregnant condition and to appreciate fully all feasible options should be assessed. Management of the pregnant patient with a psychotic disorder should first be directed toward stabilization of her psychiatric condition. For patients whose condition presents a danger to either themselves or their unborn babies, it is invariably necessary to institute involuntary hospitalization. Collateral support from the partner and family members should be elicited. Once the patient's condition is stabilized, management issues related to continuation or termination of the pregnancy can be addressed.

# Pregnancy Loss

When intrauterine death involves a fetus of up to 20 weeks gestational age, the event is called a spontaneous abortion (miscarriage). Between 20 and 37 weeks gestational age, the loss of a fetus is considered a preterm birth. When an infant is lost after 37 weeks' gestation, a stillbirth is said to have occurred.

## Epidemiology and Etiology of Pregnancy Loss

Of recognized pregnancies, 12%–24% result in miscarriage (Lee and Slade 1996). Because up to one-third of all miscarriages are unrecognized, the rate is probably much higher, perhaps up to 50%. Most pregnancy losses occur within the first 3 months of pregnancy. Of reproductive-age couples, 1% experience three or more consecutive miscarriages.

More than 60% of early fetal losses are thought to be due to fetal defects (Frost and Condon 1996). Maternal or unknown factors account for the remaining early losses, although in some cases early loss may be due to more than one factor. Later losses are usually the result of maternal factors (e.g., hypertension, cervical incompetence, diabetes) that result in preterm delivery of a nonviable fetus. The rise in tubal pregnancies, which is responsible for 2% of pregnancy losses in the United States, is thought to be due to the increased incidence of pelvic inflammatory disease, tubal complications resulting from intrauterine devices and gynecological surgeries, and smoking (Attar 2004; Stone 1995).

## Perceptions of Pregnancy Loss

Perhaps as a reaction to the frequent occurrence of miscarriage, lay and medical communities have traditionally viewed pregnancy loss (particularly in the first trimester) as a relatively minor event. The event is generally not associated with culturally accepted rituals such as a burial, a memorial service, or condolence cards. Friends and family frequently try to alleviate the sorrow of the grieving couple with comments such as "it's just as well because there was probably something wrong with the baby anyway" or "you can always try again." Physicians, who are familiar with early pregnancy losses, tend to medicalize the event by describing it as a "blighted ovum" or fetal demise. Such comments tend to isolate the couple, who were left to wonder whether they are capable of bearing a normal child and whether their feelings of bereavement are normal. After a miscarriage, the woman and her partner may find that they are at variance in the timing of their often intense and quickly changing feelings and may become alienated from one another.

Since the 1970s, it has been common practice to encourage the parents of a stillborn infant to see and hold their infant, with the goal of facilitating recovery from their loss and avoiding psychological sequelae for the parents. However, the findings of a small study have called this practice into question (Hughes et al. 2002). In that study, women who held their stillborn infants were more depressed 1 year postpartum than those who only saw their infants, and those who did not see their infants were least likely to be depressed after 1 year. Further studies are needed to determine which of these practices is most beneficial for parents of stillborn children. At this time, it is probably best to offer but not insist that parents see and hold their dead infant.

## Dynamic Aspects of Pregnancy Loss

Although a primary outcome of a healthy pregnancy is the birth of a healthy baby, pregnancy also has a number of meanings that are related to the enhancement of self-esteem. Establishing biological continuity over generations bolsters one's sense of power, affirms gender identity, and assuages anxiety associated with fears of death (Leon 1992). Because a miscarriage occurs just as a woman has entered a transition involving the creation of life, fetal loss is frequently experienced as personal failure. Just as she is preparing to progress through a new developmental stage, the woman who has sustained a perinatal loss is faced with a developmental obstacle.

### Psychological Sequelae After Pregnancy Loss

Women who experience a pregnancy loss exhibit more anxiety, depression, and somatization in the 6 months after the event than do women who have successfully delivered healthy babies (Janssen et al. 1996; Neugebauer et al. 1997). At particular risk for major depression are women who are childless or who have a history of major depression. Severity of postmiscarriage depression is greater with younger age and higher numbers of prior reproductive losses (Neugebauer 2003). A history of major depression places a woman at more than a 50% risk of experiencing a recurrent episode of depression after perinatal loss (Neugebauer et al. 1997). The depression usually begins within the first month after miscarriage and tends to diminish with time, so that by the end of 1 year significant mental distress is unusual. Many women who experience an intrauterine loss become pregnant and deliver a healthy baby by 1 year after the initial loss.

In one study, women who had experienced a prior *late* fetal death (after 18 weeks' gestation) and who became pregnant within a year were significantly more likely to be depressed and anxious in the third trimester of their next pregnancy and at 1 year postpartum (Hughes et al. 1999). However, women who waited at least 1 year after the fetal loss before becoming pregnant again were no more likely than a control group to experience depression or anxiety. Whether this outcome occurs because women who experience late-term intrauterine loss need a year to allow for mourning before beginning another pregnancy or because women who choose to conceive sooner are more vulnerable to depression and anxiety is a subject for further study. However, it may be prudent for women and their partners who have suffered a late-term pregnancy loss to wait 12 months before attempting conception.

### Treatment Recommendations

Couples who have sustained a pregnancy loss need to work through their bereavement in a safe place where fears can be discussed, disappointments addressed, and grief experienced. For couples who are feeling isolated and alienated, the psychiatrist may be able to provide an opportunity for such processes to occur. The consultation should include a full psychiatric assessment of the woman and her partner. It is important to distinguish psychopathology from normal bereavement. Psychiatric history should be noted carefully, and particularly close follow-up should be ensured for patients who have a history of depression or have experienced late-trimester fetal loss. Under no circumstances is prolonged disabling depression a normal grief reaction. Even if character pathology is noted, the loss of a fetus generally precludes any attempts at effecting personality change during the therapy after the loss. Psychotherapy can be time-limited and focused around the loss and its meaning to the patient and her partner. Treatment should be multimodal, utilizing elements of supportive psychotherapy to encourage healthy defenses, cognitive-behavioral therapy to diminish phobic responses to traumatic stimuli, and interpersonal therapy to sort out interpersonal behaviors that impede empathic communication.

Patients frequently sense when they are ready to leave therapy, but they should be encouraged to call if they experience recurrent depression or anxiety after discontinuing therapy. If the grief response persists, worsens, or develops into a major depression or other Axis I disorder, pharmacotherapy should be considered. If the woman and her partner decide that they would like to try to become pregnant again, the choice of medication management should include a risk-benefit analysis of medication use during pregnancy and the postpartum period. The risks and benefits should be carefully discussed in therapy, particularly because these patients are likely to be extremely cautious about using any medication that might jeopardize a subsequent pregnancy. Because women with a history of depression may be at risk for depression and anxiety during the next pregnancy, the psychiatrist should offer to resume therapy once conception occurs.

# References

Attar E: Endocrinology of ectopic pregnancy. Obstet Gynecol Clin North Am 31:779–794, x, 2004

Christiansen M, Larsen SO, Oxvig C, et al: Screening for Down's syndrome in early and late first and second trimester using six maternal serum markers. Clin Genet 65:11–16, 2004

Dagg PK: The psychological sequelae of therapeutic abortion—denied and completed. Am J Psychiatry 148:578–585, 1991

Frank PI, Kay CR, Scott LM, et al: Pregnancy following induced abortion: maternal morbidity, congenital abnormalities and neonatal death. Br J Obstet Gynaecol 94:836–842, 1987

Frost M, Condon JT: The psychological sequelae of miscarriage: a critical review of the literature. Aust N Z J Psychiatry 30:54–62, 1996

Grimes DA, Creinin MD: Induced abortion: an overview for internists. Ann Intern Med 140:620–626, 2004

Henshaw SK, Silverman J: The characteristics and prior contraceptive use of U.S. abortion patients. Fam Plann Perspect 20:158–168, 1988

Hern WM: Abortion Practice (reprint). Boulder, CO, Alpenglo Graphics, 1990

Hughes PM, Turton P, Evans CD: Stillbirth as risk factor for depression and anxiety in the subsequent pregnancy: cohort study. BMJ 318:1721–1724, 1999

Hughes P, Turton P, Hopper E, et al: Assessment of guidelines for good practice in psychosocial care of mothers after stillbirth: a cohort study. Lancet 360:114–118, 2002

Janssen HJ, Cuisinier MC, Hoogduin KA, et al: Controlled prospective study on the mental health of women following pregnancy loss. Am J Psychiatry 153:226–230, 1996

Lee C, Slade P: Miscarriage as a traumatic event: a review of the literature and new implications for intervention. J Psychosom Res 40:235–244, 1996

Leon IG: The psychoanalytic conceptualization of perinatal loss: a multidimensional model. Am J Psychiatry 149:1464–1472, 1992

Major B, Cozzarelli C, Cooper ML, et al: Psychological responses of women after first-trimester abortion. Arch Gen Psychiatry 57:777–784, 2000

Neugebauer R: Depressive symptoms at two months after miscarriage: interpreting study findings from an epidemiological versus clinical perspective. Depress Anxiety 17:152–162, 2003

Neugebauer R, Kline J, Shrout P, et al: Major depressive disorder in the 6 months after miscarriage. JAMA 277:383–388, 1997

Speckhard A, Rue VM: Postabortion syndrome: an emerging public health concern. J Soc Issues 48:95–120, 1992

Stone LR: Pregnancy losses, in Primary Care of Women. Edited by Lemcke DP, Pattison J, Marshall LA, et al. Norwalk, CT, Appleton & Lange, 1995, pp 531–539

Stotland NL: Induced abortion in the United States, in Psychological Aspects of Women's Health Care: The Interface Between Psychiatry and Obstetrics and Gynecology, 2nd Edition. Edited by Stotland NL, Stewart DE. Washington, DC, American Psychiatric Press, 2001, pp 219–239

Stotland NL: Psychiatric issues related to infertility, reproductive technologies, and abortion. Prim Care 29:13–26, v, 2002

Strauss LT, Herndon J, Chang J, et al: Abortion surveillance—United States, 2001. MMWR Surveill Summ 53(9):1–32, 2004

Westfall JM, O'Brien-Gonzales A, Barley G: Update on early medical and surgical abortion. J Womens Health 7:991–995, 1998

Westhoff C, Picardo L, Morrow E: Quality of life following early medical or surgical abortion. Contraception 67:41–47, 2003

Zolese G, Blacker CV: The psychological complications of therapeutic abortion. Br J Psychiatry 160:742–749, 1992

# 7

# Infertility

## Psychological Implications of Diagnosis and Treatment

## Epidemiology

Infertility is defined as the inability of a couple to achieve pregnancy after at least 1 year of unprotected intercourse. In the United States, approximately 10%–15% of all couples experience infertility (Evers 2002). The number of women known to have a fertility problem increased from 4.9 million in 1988 to 6.2 million in 1995, and about 44% of those sought medical help. The cost of infertility treatment is substantial, particularly for assisted reproductive technologies (i.e., techniques involving direct retrieval of oocytes from the ovary) (Gleicher 2000). Approximately 50% of infertile couples eventually conceive.

## Etiology

Infertility may be secondary to a male factor, a female factor, or a combination of factors contributed by both members of a couple (Table 7–1). Historically, women were thought to bear the sole responsibility for infertility; now it is believed that male factors contribute to 40%–60% of infertility (Adamson and Baker 2003; Stephen and Chandra 1998). In 10%–30% of couples, two or more factors cause the infertility (Adamson and Baker 2003; Stephen and

**Table 7–1.**    Causes of infertility

| Source of problem | % |
| --- | --- |
| Male factor | 40–60 |
| Ovarian factor | 30 |
| Disease of uterus or fallopian tubes | 20 |
| Cervical factor, immunological factors, infection | 5 |
| Unknown | 20 |

Chandra 1998). Up to 10% of cases of infertility may be partially or completely explained by premature ejaculation and impotence (Seibel and Taymor 1982). Psychological factors contributing to infertility include anorexia nervosa and stress-induced amenorrhea. Recent data suggest that having a history of depression or being currently depressed may be associated with a decline in ovarian function (Harlow et al. 2003).

# Related Psychological Factors

For most couples, infertility is a significant life crisis. Infertile couples pass through a series of phases, including disbelief, denial, frustration, anger, grief, and eventually acceptance. For couples who choose to undergo treatment, huge monetary costs add to the stress they experience. Although infertility clearly affects the marital relationship, it may strengthen some couples' relationships, possibly because of the shared experience and participation in treating the problem.

## Psychological Factors for the Woman

Infertile women tend to feel frustrated and less feminine and to experience decreased self-esteem (Anderson et al. 2003). Women experiencing infertility report high levels of psychological distress, dysphoria, a decline in their sexual functioning, and a feeling of lowered self-worth. In many cases, infertile women feel that the issue of their infertility has become so all-important to them that they are less interested in other aspects of their lives (Anderson et al. 2003).

When a couple is faced with infertility, women tend to be more emotionally affected than their male partners (Anderson et al. 2003). This tendency appears at the point of the initial diagnosis and continues even after years of treatment.

## Psychological Factors for the Man

Some men experience considerable anxiety while undergoing infertility evaluation and treatment, either because the infertility results in part or fully from a male factor or because the treatment requires performance by the man in a scheduled manner. Particularly for men with anxious personalities, the demands of sexual performance during the fertile portion of the woman's menstrual cycle make it difficult or impossible to sustain an erection. It may also be difficult for men to produce a semen sample for the postcoital examination or for intrauterine insemination. For men, as for women, self-esteem is often closely connected to the ability to perform sexually.

## Psychological Factors Shared by the Couple

Infertile couples often feel socially isolated, particularly when their peers are occupied with child rearing and organize their social activities around their children. In an effort to avoid painful questioning about their childlessness or future plans, such couples may avoid family gatherings. The financial burden of both evaluation and treatment for infertility is an additional significant source of stress and may mean alterations in financial decisions, such as purchasing a home or a car or taking vacations. Not uncommonly, couples will turn to the use of credit cards to finance expensive technological approaches, even when the likelihood of their success is poor. Infertile women undergoing assisted reproductive technological treatment may postpone or refuse career advancement opportunities because of the physical and logistical demands entailed by the treatment.

# Evaluation

The assessment for infertility is both comprehensive and extensive and often involves evaluation of both partners (Table 7–2). It includes baseline evaluations of general health and use of medications and substances (e.g., alcohol, recreational drugs) that may impair fertility, screening for sexually transmit-

**Table 7–2.**    Diagnostic studies to evaluate infertility

Comprehensive medical, surgical, reproductive history of both partners

Physical examination of both partners

Endocrine evaluations for both partners

Basal body temperature charting in the woman; recording of dates of intercourse

Semen analysis

Postcoital test

Endometrial biopsy

Hysterosalpingogram

Laparoscopy

Tests of patency of male ductile system

ted diseases and normal endocrine functioning, assessment of ovulation, assessment of the quantity and quality of sperm, visualization of the woman's anatomy, and determination of the patency of ductile systems in the woman and/or the man. Tests are often repeated at intervals over a single menstrual cycle and at subsequent menstrual cycles. The assessment invariably requires substantial reorganization of the day-to-day lives of both partners, because office visits are dictated by responses to treatment, dates of ovulation, and physicians' schedules.

One of the first studies frequently included in an infertility assessment is daily basal body temperature recording for at least 1 or 2 months. Each morning before rising, the woman records her body temperature. A temperature rise occurs in response to ovulation and the increase in the level of progesterone. The days when intercourse has occurred are also recorded. Another early study, the postcoital test, involves a sampling of cervical mucus collected from the woman within 8 hours after intercourse. The couple is instructed not to have intercourse for 1–2 days before the sampling. The sample is then assayed for its suitability as an environment for sperm and for the quantity and quality of motile sperm. Although these diagnostic tests appear rather simple, they involve sharing the details of sexual acts with medical personnel, who often medicalize the natural and personal components of an intimate physical relationship. Men frequently have performance anxiety, and both men and women may feel frustrated, irritable, anxious, and angry.

Early in the evaluation for infertility, the man collects semen by masturbation. Although technically simple, the process is difficult for many men, who are sometimes unable to perform on command in the setting of a medical office. The semen is analyzed microscopically to confirm adequate volume, viscosity, pH, sperm count, motility, and morphology and to rule out infectious agents such as *Ureaplasma* and *Mycoplasma*. Oligospermia, or low sperm count, varies from mild (sperm concentration of 5–20 million/mL) to severe (under 1 million/mL). Asthenospermia, or abnormal sperm motility, is diagnosed if fewer than 50% of sperm are motile, and teratospermia refers to sperm with morphological abnormalities in over 85% of the sample (Iammarrone et al. 2003).

For the woman whose cervical mucus appears to be normal and who is ovulating regularly but is nevertheless unable to conceive, a hysterosalpingogram is often performed. This examination, which visualizes any mechanical blockage to sperm, involves the injection of radiopaque dye into the female reproductive tract. The woman may experience a side effect of transient pelvic cramping. Laparoscopy, involving direct visualization of the female reproductive organs by insertion of a laparoscope through the navel (with the patient under general anesthesia), may also be performed to rule out anatomic abnormalities.

## Treatment of Infertility

Whenever possible, infertility treatment is aimed at reversing pathology isolated by assessment studies (see Table 7–3). When hysterosalpingography or laparoscopy reveals mechanical blockage or anatomical abnormalities (present in 40%–50% of cases of female infertility), treatment is directed at removing the defect. In some cases, adhesions from endometriosis may be removed by means of a laparoscopic procedure. Gonadotropin-releasing hormone (GnRH) agonists such as leuprolide acetate, goserelin, and nafarelin acetate are the treatments of choice for endometriosis. Any of these treatments may cause depression or emotional lability.

In cases of ovulatory dysfunction, induction of ovulation is attempted initially with orally administered clomiphene citrate, a nonsteroidal antiestrogen. Potential psychiatric side effects of clomiphene citrate include depression, nervousness, and insomnia. If, after several attempts, ovulation has not been successfully induced by clomiphene citrate, human menopausal gona-

**Table 7–3.** Current treatment of infertility

| Cause of infertility | Treatment |
| --- | --- |
| Ovulatory dysfunction | Clomiphene citrate, gonadotropin |
| Tubal injury, blockage, or destruction | Surgical repair |
| Male factor | Donor or intrauterine insemination |
| Endometriosis | Ablation |
| Cervical factor | Intrauterine insemination |
| Luteal-phase deficiency | Progesterone or clomiphene citrate |
| Unexplained | Clomiphene citrate, gonadotropin, intrauterine insemination |

dotropins may be administered by daily injections. (Medications used include menotropins, a combination of follicle-stimulating hormone and luteinizing hormone, and urofollitropin.) Injections may be performed by the woman herself or her partner, or she may want to make daily visits to her physician for administration of the drug. Side effects may include fatigue, nausea, headache, diarrhea, and weight gain. The likelihood of multiple gestation (usually twins) is increased to 5% with clomiphene citrate and 20% with human menopausal gonadotropins. The administration of pulsatile GnRH through a portable infusion pump is an alternative that produces a lower rate of multiple gestation (Tan et al. 1996), but this strategy is not widely available. Throughout the procedure, serial ultrasounds are used to confirm normal ovulation and monitor follicular development. Pharmacological induction of ovulation is more likely to be successful if combined with intrauterine insemination. The success rate of these two combined procedures currently approximates 33% (Guzick et al. 1999).

When infertility persists after conventional therapy, or when fallopian tubes are irreversibly obstructed or damaged, infertile couples are treated with assisted reproductive technology (Table 7–4). This term includes techniques that involve retrieving oocytes directly from the ovary. Embryos or gametes are then transferred directly into the woman. Ovulation is induced by injections of gonadotropin, and oocytes are retrieved. In gamete intrafallopian transfer (GIFT), oocytes and sperm are immediately placed in the fallopian tubes. In zygote intrafallopian transfer (ZIFT), fertilized embryos are placed in the tubes 1–2 days after retrieval. For in vitro fertilization (IVF), fertilized

**Table 7–4.** Success rates for assisted reproductive technology cycles using fresh nondonor eggs or embryos

| Measure | Success rate (%) |
| --- | --- |
| Pregnancies per cycle | 34.3 |
| Live births per cycle | 28.3 |
| Live births per retrieval | 32.6 |
| Live births per transfer | 34.8 |
| Singleton live births per cycle | 21.1 |
| Singleton live births per transfer | 22.5 |

*Source.* Assisted reproductive technology success rates: national summary and fertility clinic reports, 2002. Atlanta, GA, Centers for Disease Control and Prevention, Division of Reproductive Health. Available at: www.cdc.gov/reproductivehealth/ART02/index.htm.

embryos are placed directly into the uterine cavity. Serial ultrasounds are administered and estradiol levels are assayed to monitor ovulation and posttransfer development and to rule out ovarian hyperstimulation. These procedures are exceedingly expensive—thousands of dollars per attempt—and most couples are advised to make three to four attempts. Because multiple gametes or zygotes are often transferred at one time, assisted reproductive technology increases the probability of multiple gestation to about 25%. There is also a 6% chance of severe ovarian hyperstimulation syndrome, a potentially life-threatening complication. Intracytoplasmic sperm injection (ICSI)—in which a tiny pipette is used to inject a single sperm into the egg—followed by artificial insemination is used for severe male factor infertility.

In an analysis of registry data for births over a 4-year period in western Australia, Hansen et al. (2002) found that infants conceived with assisted reproductive technology (either intracytoplasmic sperm injection or IVF) may be more than twice as likely as naturally conceived infants to have major birth defects and also are more likely to have multiple major defects. This finding was true for both singletons and multiple-gestation infants (Hansen et al. 2002). Furthermore, a large study revealed that the use of assisted reproductive technology appears to be associated with an increased risk of low-birthweight infants both for singletons and multiple-gestation infants (Schieve et al. 2002). In this study, infants conceived with assisted reproductive technology accounted for 0.6% of all infants born in the United States to mothers

20 years of age or older, but for 3.5% of low-birth-weight and 4.3% of very-low-birth-weight infants. The use of assisted reproductive technology therefore seems to double the risk of having a singleton with low birth weight or a child with a major birth defect. Nevertheless, in absolute terms, 94% of couples who require reproductive assistance and succeed in having a single baby will have a normal-birth-weight infant, and 91% will have an infant free of major birth defects (Mitchell 2002). For many infertile couples, the low risk of having small infants with a birth defect may make the procedure acceptable. However, the number of IVF procedures increased by 37% between 1995 and 1998, and it has been speculated that this increase is a direct result of increased marketing of assisted reproductive services, which tends to encourage the use of these procedures by couples who might be able to conceive naturally if they waited longer before requesting consultation. The risks of assisted reproductive technology should therefore be carefully reviewed by all couples before they proceed with treatment (Mitchell 2002).

When infertility is due to a male factor that is not treatable, artificial insemination by a donor (AID), also called therapeutic donor insemination (TDI), is a technically simple and highly successful modality. Receiving a donated egg is a useful strategy for the woman who is unable to ovulate even with medical assistance. This process is more complex than AID, because it involves treatment of the donor and the infertile woman with medications to synchronize their cycles. By means of IVF or GIFT, donor eggs are fertilized with sperm and the infertile woman is inseminated and carries the pregnancy. A more controversial treatment involves the use of a surrogate mother to carry the fertilized egg of a woman who is able to ovulate but not to carry a pregnancy successfully.

Many women who undergo infertility treatment are over age 35 years and therefore face higher risks of having a child with a chromosomal abnormality such as Down syndrome and trisomy 18. A new technique, referred to as first trimester prenatal screening, combines an ultrasound examination of the fluid accumulation behind the neck of the fetus (nuchal translucency) and a blood test for levels of free β-human chorionic gonadotropin (β-HCG) and pregnancy associated plasma protein A (PAPP-A). This procedure allows for tentative diagnoses of chromosomal abnormalities and other conditions as early as the 11th week of pregnancy (Snijders and Smith 2002). If the test shows an increased risk of a chromosomal abnormality, the woman is referred for further testing, including chorionic villus sampling and/or amniocentesis.

# Psychological Reactions to Infertility Treatment

Infertility treatment—with its stresses of constantly monitoring reproduction-related bodily functions, regulating intimate sexual acts, and spending large sums of money with no guarantee of success—places the couple at risk for dysphoria and anxiety (Table 7–5). Also, many of the medications used in infertility treatment protocols can produce side effects such as moodiness and irritability. Mood swings also occur as a reaction to the stress of pursuing conception over the course of many months.

**Table 7–5.**   Adverse effects of infertility and infertility procedures

Depression, anxiety, hostility (more common in women than in men)
Negative effect on sexual functioning: impotence, anorgasmia, decreased libido
Social isolation
Financial difficulties
Unrealistic expectations of outcome of pregnancy
Multiple births

Partners often find that in synchronizing their sexual acts with the needs of the fertility treatment, the spontaneity of their sexual relationship is lost. This loss may result in an inability to perform on the part of either the man, who may be unable to maintain an erection or to ejaculate, or the woman, who may suffer from vaginismus or dyspareunia. If multiple gestation occurs, there is an increased risk of premature births and of medical problems in the infants; this frequently contributes to additional stress on the couple. Often, when a couple has been infertile for a number of years and has been single-mindedly devoted to achieving pregnancy through assisted reproductive technology, little thought is given to the realities of child rearing. Paradoxically, such couples may be faced with a letdown when they achieve their goal of becoming parents.

Women who have postponed childbearing to accomplish career aspirations are often used to maintaining control over their lives and achieving carefully planned goals. When these women discover that they are unsuccessful at achieving pregnancy, they may feel frustrated and angry because they are now faced with a situation over which they have no control. Guilt because of conscious past decisions to postpone conception or to undergo prior therapeutic abortions is not uncommon.

## Treatment of Psychological Difficulties Related to Infertility

Frequently, infertility specialists refer an infertile woman for psychiatric assessment before beginning or continuing her treatment for infertility. For patients who have undergone continuous treatment without success, a treatment holiday may be helpful to allow a couple to return to a more natural routine without the dictates of medical intervention. This holiday period also allows time to reevaluate alternative options. Even if one member of a couple is more disabled psychiatrically than the other, it is often very helpful to see both members of the couple for at least several sessions. RESOLVE, the national self-help organization for infertile couples, sponsors support groups throughout the United States that are often very helpful in destigmatizing the issue of infertility and enabling couples to feel both strengthened and less isolated (See Appendix).

Although infertile women are no more likely to develop a major depressive disorder or anxiety disorder than are women in the general population, in some cases the stress of diagnosis and treatment may cause or exacerbate psychiatric disorders. For mild to moderate psychiatric symptoms, psychotherapy may be all that is necessary. Group psychological interventions can be effective and have been reported to increase pregnancy rates in infertile women (Domar et al. 2000). For major mood or anxiety disorders, treatment should involve psychotherapy and/or psychotropic medication. The use of medications to induce ovulation or sustain gestation may complicate treatment, because many of these agents may exacerbate psychiatric difficulties or reduce the effectiveness of psychotropic medications. Collaborative discussions should include the psychiatrist, the couple, and the treating infertility specialist. The psychiatrist may provide a supportive environment in which the couple can realistically review the probability of achieving success with further infertility treatments. Empathic psychotherapy to explore alternative options, including postponement of infertility treatments, adoption, and ways other than parenting to derive gratification for caregiving aspirations, may also be helpful. Should the couple decide to move ahead with further infertility treatments, the psychiatrist may then provide ongoing support and treatment (Table 7–6).

**Table 7–6.**   Roles for psychiatry in the treatment of infertility

Performing a psychiatric evaluation

Helping patients to clarify issues, gain insight into motivations, make choice that best serves their interests

Helping patients with decision making

Helping partners reach consensus

Helping patients cope with stresses of infertility treatments

Providing treatment holidays

Referring patients for individual supportive therapy

Referring patients to support groups (see Appendix)

Providing psychopharmacological treatment

# When the Infertile Couple Succeeds in Achieving Pregnancy

For the couple whose energy has been focused for years on the achievement of a successful impregnation, the realization of a long-awaited child is invariably met with great joy and relief. It is not unusual, however, for the previously infertile couple to encounter significant difficulties with their new roles as parents. In trying to achieve pregnancy, the couple may have neglected to anticipate their roles as parents of a child whose presence means renegotiating their relationship with each other. In addition, as a woman's body grows over the 9 months of pregnancy, the couple's triumph after the long years during which they felt inadequate in comparison with their peers may be so great that they have difficulty in letting go of the increasingly visible pregnant state.

For many infertile couples who have been in psychotherapy, it is therefore helpful to continue in psychotherapy over the course of pregnancy and through at least the first 6 months of parenthood. In a supportive psychotherapeutic setting, both partners will have the opportunity to explore their relationship apart from issues related to fertility, sexual performance on command, or connections with medical personnel. Reevaluating the emotional bonds that connected them long before they were aware of fertility difficulties may be important for the couple as they await and anticipate the birth of their child.

# References

Adamson GD, Baker VL: Subfertility: causes, treatment and outcome. Best Pract Res Clin Obstet Gynaecol 17:169–85, 2003

Anderson KM, Sharpe M, Rattray A, et al: Distress and concerns in couples referred to a specialist infertility clinic. J Psychosom Res 54:353–355, 2003

Domar AD, Clapp D, Slawsby EA, et al: Impact of group psychological interventions on pregnancy rates in infertile women. Fertil Steril 73:805–811, 2000

Evers JL: Female subfertility. Lancet 360:151–159, 2002

Gleicher N: Cost-effective infertility care. Hum Reprod Update 6:190–199, 2000

Guzick DS, Carson SA, Coutifaris C, et al: Efficacy of superovulation and intrauterine insemination in the treatment of infertility. National Cooperative Reproductive Medicine Network. N Engl J Med 340:177–183, 1999

Hansen M, Kurinczuk JJ, Bower C, et al: The risk of major birth defects after intracytoplasmic sperm injection and in vitro fertilization. N Engl J Med 346:725–730, 2002

Harlow BL, Wise LA, Otto MW, et al: Depression and its influence on reproductive endocrine and menstrual cycle markers associated with perimenopause: the Harvard Study of Moods and Cycles. Arch Gen Psychiatry 60:29–36, 2003

Iammarrone E, Balet R, Lower AM, et al: Male infertility. Best Pract Res Clin Obstet Gynaecol 17:211–229, 2003

Mitchell AA: Infertility treatment—more risks and challenges. N Engl J Med 346:769–770, 2002

Schieve LA, Miekle SF, Ferre C, et al: Low and very low birth weight in infants conceived with use of assisted reproductive technology. N Engl J Med 346:731–737, 2002

Seibel MM, Taymor ML: Emotional aspects of infertility. Fertil Steril 37:137–145, 1982

Snijders R, Smith E: The role of fetal nuchal translucency in prenatal screening. Curr Opin Obstet Gynecol 14:577–585, 2002

Stephen EH, Chandra A: Updated projections of infertility in the United States, 1995–2025. Fertil Steril 70:30–34, 1998

Tan SL, Farhi J, Homburg R, et al: Induction of ovulation in clomiphene-resistant polycystic ovary syndrome with pulsatile GnRH. Obstet Gynecol 88:221–226, 1996

# 8

# Perimenopause and Menopause

## Definitions and History

Menopause is the point at which a woman has permanently ceased menstruating. Perimenopause, which typically occurs 5–7 years before menopause, is the interval between regular ovulatory menstrual cycles and complete cessation of ovarian function. The term *climacteric* derives from the Greek word for rung of a ladder and describes the years of declining ovarian function corresponding to the passage from the reproductive to the nonreproductive phases of life.

Until recently, menopause was thought to be a time of moodiness, irritability, and somatization. In 1890, Kraepelin coined the term *involutional melancholia* for a syndrome of agitated depression, hypochondriasis, and nihilistic delusions. This syndrome was included as a diagnostic category in DSM-I (American Psychiatric Association 1952) and DSM-II (American Psychiatric Association 1968). Because extensive epidemiological data collected in the 1970s found no evidence for the diagnosis, it was dropped from DSM-III (American Psychiatric Association 1980).

Natural menopause occurs between the ages of 44 and 55 years (average = 51.4 years). Because women in the United States now live to an average age of 81 years, the postmenopausal years often constitute more than one-third of a woman's life. In addition to experiencing physiological changes during the perimenopausal and menopausal years, some women experience mood alterations.

## Hormonal Changes

During perimenopause, when ovarian function and fertility are declining, there may be few signs of this reproductive transition. The interval between menstrual periods may shorten or lengthen, and menstrual bleeding may become lighter or heavier. Occasionally a period is skipped, and this event generally corresponds to a month when ovulation has not occurred. As menopause is approached, menstrual periods become progressively lighter and more infrequent, and then cease completely.

Menopause has been presumed to be solely a response to ovarian failure. Thus, in response to decreased estrogen production by the ovary, the levels of two pituitary hormones—luteinizing hormone (LH) and follicle-stimulating hormone (FSH)—rise. The ovarian hormone inhibin, which negatively feeds back to decrease FSH release, also decreases and is thought to also contribute to the rise in FSH. Recent data from the Study of Women's Health Across the Nation (SWAN), an observational project, suggest that menopause may rather result from a relative hypothalamic-pituitary insensitivity to estrogen (Weiss et al. 2004). An elevated serum FSH level, measured on the second or third day after the onset of menses, suggests a woman is perimenopausal. Elevated FSH levels obtained later in the cycle can be misleading because the level of this hormone may rise into the menopausal range in premenopausal women, particularly at midcycle (Figure 2–2). At and after menopause, levels of estradiol, the biologically active form of estrogen, remain below 25 pg/mL, and levels of FSH remain above 40 mIU/mL.

Circulating levels of steroids are determined largely by ovarian steroid production, peripheral conversion of steroids to their active forms, and concentrations of sex hormone–binding globulin (SHBG). After menopause, the estradiol-producing ovarian follicles undergo atresia, but the androgen-producing thecal/interstitial cells of the ovaries continue to produce testosterone and androstenedione. Estrogen production in postmenopausal women is mainly in the form of estrone resulting from peripheral aromatization of adrenal and ovarian androstenedione. By binding to hormones, SHBG reduces the concentrations of free, or biologically active, androgens and estrogens. Androgens in turn reduce SHBG concentrations, whereas estrogens increase them. Postmenopause, the concentration of SHBG decreases slightly. Treatment with exogenous estrogen increases SHBG and therefore reduces free serum testosterone (Shifren and Schiff 2000).

# Physical Changes

The physical signs and symptoms of perimenopause and menopause result from declining estrogen production. Vasomotor symptoms, including hot flashes and cold sweats, occur in 80% of perimenopausal women. These symptoms may persist for several years beyond the last menstrual period. Hot flashes are sensations of extreme heat that develop unexpectedly in the face, upper body, or entire body and last for 1–5 minutes. They are followed by sweating and a feeling of cold as perspiration evaporates. Breathlessness, dizziness, and an increased heart rate may occur. Because these symptoms are not unlike those of panic attacks, the differential diagnosis of new-onset panic disorder in the middle-aged woman should include perimenopausal vasomotor symptoms. When vasomotor symptoms occur at night, a woman may experience insomnia and the subsequent effects of sleep deprivation, including decreased concentration, fatigue, and irritability. Hot flashes often occur when women are still menstruating.

The decline in ovarian estrogen production is associated with a number of physical changes, including atrophy of the urogenital tract lining, sometimes resulting in inflammation of the vagina and urinary tract. Infection and dyspareunia (painful intercourse) may result, with subsequent urinary frequency, urgency, and occasional stress incontinence. Osteoporosis and urogenital atrophy are long-term consequences of low estrogen levels.

# Mood Changes

## Natural Menopause

In general, longitudinal studies have not found that natural menopause increases the risk for depression in most women (Kaufert et al. 1992). However, some women may experience depression during the perimenopause. In particular, women who experience a lengthy perimenopause appear to be at risk for depressive symptoms. Two very large prospective epidemiological studies that included more than 12,000 subjects have shown that as women pass from premenopause to postmenopause, they are at increased risk for depression (Bromberger et al. 2001; Maartens et al. 2002). Data from a recent 4-year prospective study of more than 300 premenopausal women indicated that depressive symptoms increased during the transition to menopause and decreased after menopause, even after adjustment for other predictors of depression, including a history of depression, severe premenstrual syndrome (PMS), poor sleep, age, race, and employment status (Freeman et al. 2004). After menopause, mood symptoms often return to baseline. The same study indicated that the faster the rise in FSH (i.e., the shorter the perimenopausal transition), the less likely were subjects to experience depression. Other risk factors for perimenopausal depression are a history of depression, including postpartum depression, a history of severe PMS, poor sleep, being unemployed, financial problems, death of a partner, death of a child, and the presence of hot flashes (Freeman et al. 2004; Maartens et al. 2002). Data from an earlier large prospective general population study indicated that besides a history of depression, health problems and social stressors also increase the risk of depressive symptoms in perimenopausal women. The risk for perimenopausal depression is also increased by being divorced, widowed, or separated; having a lower level of education; and experiencing stress from caretaking responsibilities (Avis and McKinlay 1991, 1995). It is interesting to note that neither the death of parents nor the experience of children leaving the home seems to be a risk factor for the development of depression at menopause (Kaufert et al. 1992). Depression in women before perimenopause increases the likelihood of depression during the perimenopausal years (Table 8–1).

**Table 8–1.**    Factors implicated in perimenopausal depression

Lengthy perimenopause (slower rise in follicle-stimulating hormone)

History of depression, including postpartum depression

History of severe premenstrual syndrome

Hot flashes

Sleep problems

Chronic health problems

Loss of significant other (death of a partner, divorce, separation, death of a child)

Caretaking responsibilities

Financial problems

Unemployment

Lower level of education

## Surgical Menopause

A total hysterectomy involves removal of the uterus, whereas a total hysterectomy with bilateral salpingoophorectomy refers to removal of the uterus and ovaries. For many women who undergo either of these procedures to relieve severe symptoms such as menorrhagia, pelvic pain, and severe PMS, psychological functioning tends to improve after surgery. However, women with psychiatric histories are more likely to experience adverse psychological reactions after a hysterectomy (Khastgir et al. 2000). Other risk factors for poor psychiatric outcome after hysterectomy include having the hysterectomy at a young age, undergoing the procedure emergently rather than electively, having poor social supports, experiencing marital dysfunction, having a low socioeconomic status, and having a history of multiple surgeries (Hillard 1993) (Table 8–2). Preoperative preparation should be directed toward addressing negative expectations of the effects of surgery as well as understanding and appreciating the emotional meaning of the surgery to the patient. For patients experiencing depression or other psychiatric conditions before surgery, it is particularly important to treat the psychiatric condition before the surgery and, if possible, to delay surgery until a good treatment response is attained. Psychiatric follow-up after the hysterectomy is helpful to ensure psychiatric stability.

**Table 8–2.**  Factors implicated in postsurgical menopausal depression

History of depression
Young age
Poor social supports
Marital dysfunction
Lower socioeconomic status
History of multiple surgeries
Surgery performed emergently

For premenopausal women who undergo a procedure involving the removal of both uterus and ovaries, one outcome is a precipitous drop in estrogen level. These women almost invariably experience hot flashes, which can be particularly troublesome and may cause sleep disturbance and depression. For these women, estrogen (without progesterone) can be used to relieve vasomotor symptoms and therefore eliminate one possible cause of postoperative depressive symptoms.

## Menopause and Sexuality

### Natural Menopause

Most women who have been sexually active before menopause remain so during the perimenopausal years. Nevertheless, estrogen decline associated with perimenopause may produce dyspareunia and decreased libido (Dennerstein et al. 2001). It appears that the level of distress arising from these changes is associated in part with lifetime sexual interest. Women who are most distressed about menopausal sexual changes are those who have had the highest sexual interest before menopause (Gelfand 2000). Atrophic urogenital tract changes that may result in vaginal dryness, infection, and subsequent dyspareunia can often be effectively treated with estrogen therapy in the form of oral supplementation, vaginal cream or vaginal estrogen rings, or skin patches. Because there are potential risks (see subsection titled "Risks and Benefits" under Hormone Therapy, later in this chapter) associated with long-term use of systemic estrogen, estrogen therapy in the form of a local vaginal cream or ring is generally considered to be preferable for treatment of urogenital atrophic changes. For women whose main symptom is diminished libido, small amounts of testosterone supplementation may be helpful (Sarrel 2000; Stone and Pearlstein 1994).

Sexual dysfunction cannot always be attributed to perimenopausal urogenital changes. Other factors that may impair sexual function include diminished sexual desire, chronic health problems, depression, anxiety, medication effects, partner unavailability, relationship conflicts, or sexual dysfunction in the partner. Because elderly women often live in nursing homes or other residential facilities or live with their children, loss of privacy may also negatively affect sexual function. The assessment of sexual functioning should therefore address psychological, social, medical, and environmental issues, in addition to physical symptoms (Table 8–3).

### Surgical Menopause

Women frequently fear that hysterectomy will have a negative effect on their sexual functioning. Contrary to this view, after surgery, most women experi-

**Table 8–3.** Possible causes of sexual dysfunction in perimenopausal women

Urogenital changes (diminished vaginal lubrication, delayed clitoral reaction time, reduced vaginal blood flow, genital engorgement, dyspareunia, etc.)

Diminished sexual desire

Illness

Poor physical fitness

Depression

Anxiety

Medication effects (e.g., sexual side effects of antihypertensive agents, antipsychotics, antidepressants)

Unsatisfactory premenopausal sexual function

Partner unavailability

Relationship difficulties

Sexual dysfunction in the partner

Loss of privacy because of shared living quarters

ence improved sexual functioning (e.g., increased frequency of sexual activity and orgasm, reduction in pain during sex). This is particularly true for women who have had hysterectomies to treat dysfunctional uterine bleeding (Maas et al. 2003). Furthermore, sexual well-being tends to improve whether the surgery is a vaginal hysterectomy, subtotal hysterectomy (cervix left intact), or total abdominal hysterectomy (uterus and cervix removed) (Roovers et al. 2003). However, women who have depression before a hysterectomy tend to have poor sexual function after the procedure (Rhodes et al. 1999).

# Hormone Therapy

## Risks and Benefits

It has long been known that coronary heart disease is the leading cause of death in postmenopausal women and that osteoporosis is a widespread and disabling disease in older women. Although breast cancer is a serious, potentially lethal disease, for a 50-year-old woman, the lifetime probability of developing cardiovascular disease is almost five times greater than that of developing breast cancer (Grady et al. 1992) (Table 8–4). Until recently, on

**Table 8–4.**   Probability of breast cancer, osteoporotic hip fracture, and coronary heart disease in 50 year-old women

| Disease | Lifetime probability for a 50-year-old woman (%) | Probability of dying from disease (%) |
|---|---|---|
| Breast cancer | 10 | 3 |
| Osteoporotic hip fracture | 15 | 1.5 |
| Coronary heart disease | 46 | 31 |

*Source.*  Gelfand 2000

the basis of data gleaned from large observational studies, hormone therapy was routinely recommended for peri- and postmenopausal women to reduce the risk of fractures and heart disease. In the early to mid-1990s the Women's Health Initiative (WHI), a large randomized, placebo-controlled, prospective study of more than 27,000 healthy postmenopausal women, was instituted to study the effect of hormone therapy on the risks of coronary events, stroke, pulmonary embolism, and breast cancer. Women with an intact uterus were randomly assigned to receive estrogen plus progestin or placebo, and women without an intact uterus were randomly assigned to receive estrogen alone or placebo. In May 2002, the WHI arm of daily combined estrogen/progestin therapy was terminated early. Although this part of the study was terminated because of the increased risk of breast cancer in the hormone-therapy group, it was also found that there was an increased risk of myocardial infarction, stroke, and pulmonary embolism in subjects who received combined hormone therapy. There were also small decreases in the risks of hip fracture and colon cancer, but overall the risks outweighed the benefits of combined hormone therapy (Rossouw et al. 2002). Extrapolating from the data, the investigators reported that combined hormone therapy would result in two serious adverse events per 1,000 women treated for 1 year, and in one serious adverse event per 100 women after 5 years of treatment. More recently, results were published from the Women's Health Initiative Memory Study (WHIMS), a 6-year randomized, double-blind, placebo-controlled clinical trial involving more than 4,000 naturally postmenopausal women drawn from the larger WHI study. Data from this trial indicated that combined hormone therapy resulted in a small increased risk of dementia in treated women and provided no benefit for global cognition (Rapp et al. 2003; Shumaker et al. 2003). At the time of the termination of the combined-therapy arm of the WHI study, the adverse data did not extend to the estrogen-monotherapy arm of the study, which was permitted to continue. However, in the winter of 2004, the National Institutes of Health concluded that postmenopausal exposure to estrogen-only therapy also incurred more risks than benefits, and that trial was stopped in advance of its projected completion date of 2005. The reason for the premature termination of the estrogen-only arm of the WHI was the increased risk of stroke (Anderson et al. 2004). The data also suggested a non–statistically significant reduction in breast cancer and no effect on the risk of heart disease. Furthermore, data from the WHIMS also revealed that estrogen monotherapy increased the combined risk for dementia and mild cognitive impairment (a condition that is associated with increased risk for subsequent Alzheimer's disease) (Shumaker et al. 2004). For women age 65 years and older, estrogen monotherapy had a negative effect on global cognitive function, particularly among women whose cognitive function was lower at the inception of the study (Espeland et al. 2004). The WHIMS study group concluded that estrogen monotherapy or combined estrogen and progesterone therapy should not be initiated to protect cognitive function. Data from these studies are summarized in Table 8–5.

The results of the WHI have caused significant controversy within the medical and lay communities in the United States. Women in the study had a mean age of 63.1 years, and 85% did not experience hot flashes. Perimenopausal women, who are younger and frequently have vasomotor symptoms, were not represented in the study. Nevertheless, the data from the WHI have resulted in recommendations that extend to all women considering hormone treatment (perimenopausal and postmenopausal). The U.S. Food and Drug Administration (FDA) has advised makers of hormone therapy agents to warn potential users of the risks identified by the WHI. Combined hormonal therapies continue to be approved by the FDA for treatment of moderate-to-severe vasomotor symptoms, treatment of vulvar and vaginal atrophy, and prevention of postmenopausal osteoporosis, but treatment with the lowest dose for the shortest time is recommended to minimize associated risks.

Most clinicians agree that decisions regarding hormone therapy should be made on an individual basis and should take into consideration factors such as

**Table 8–5.** Risks and benefits of hormone therapy (estimated increase or decrease in number of events per 10,000 women in any 1 year)

| Event | Combined estrogen/ progestin therapy | Estrogen monotherapy |
|---|---|---|
| Coronary heart disease | 7 more | No effect |
| Stroke | 8 more | 12 more |
| Venous thromboembolism | 18 more | 7 more (not statistically significant for pulmonary embolism, statistically significant for deep venous thrombosis) |
| Invasive breast cancer | 8 more | 7 fewer (not statistically significant) |
| Dementia | 23 more | 12 more (not statistically significant) |
| Colorectal cancer | 6 fewer | No difference |
| Hip fracture | 5 fewer | 6 fewer |

*Note.* Unless otherwise stated, results are statistically significant.
*Source.* Anderson et al. 2004; Rossouw et al. 2002.

the woman's current health, risk for osteoporosis and cardiac disease, personal and family history of breast cancer, level of discomfort secondary to vasomotor symptoms, extent of urogenital dysfunction, and quality-of-life issues.

Certain preparations and dosages of hormones are better tolerated than others. For the 5%–10% of women who have difficulties with side effects, doses and preparations may be adjusted to minimize side effects. In some women, estrogen may cause mild breast tenderness, bloating, and headache. Side effects that have been associated with progestin include bloating, weight gain, irritability, and dysphoria (Grady et al. 1992).

Three recent controlled studies have assessed the use of estrogen for perimenopausal and postmenopausal women with major and minor depression. In two short-term treatment studies (4 weeks and 12 weeks, respectively), transdermal estrogen improved depressive symptoms in perimenopausal women

(Schmidt et al. 2000; Soares et al. 2001). In a recent preliminary 4-week study, transdermal estrogen improved depressive symptoms in six of nine perimenopausal women but only two of 11 postmenopausal women (Cohen et al. 2003). In all three studies, the mood-enhancing effect of estrogen was independent of a beneficial effect on vasomotor symptoms. Further research is needed to determine whether estrogen monotherapy will have a role in the treatment of depression in perimenopausal women. Data for estrogen as an augmenter of standard antidepressants in perimenopausal depressed women are conflicting (Amsterdam et al. 1999; Schneider et al. 1997).

## Treatment Regimens

Hormone therapy for women with an intact uterus generally requires the administration of estrogen and progestin. The progestin is prescribed to counteract the risk of endometrial cancer associated with unopposed estrogen. Hormone therapy in women who have had a hysterectomy therefore does not require a progestin in addition to estrogen.

For women with an intact uterus, hormone therapy is instituted either cyclically or continuously. Although strategies may vary among clinicians, estrogen is typically given every day of the month, and a progestin is provided either on days 1–12 of each month (cyclic regimen) or on every day of the month (continuous regimen). The advantage of the cyclic regimen is that women may reliably expect vaginal bleeding in the days after withdrawal of progestin. Bleeding at any other time of the month is unwarranted and requires gynecological assessment and endometrial biopsy to rule out endometrial hyperplasia or malignancy. The continuous regimen has the advantage of freedom from monthly bleeding, but occasional spotting may occur, particularly during the first year of hormone replacement. Endometrial biopsies may thus be required to rule out endometrial hyperplasia or malignancy.

Doses of estrogen and progestin vary with preparations (Table 8–6). In general, when an estrogen and a progestin are prescribed, doses should be as low as possible to meet treatment goals (Grady 2003).

## Testosterone and Other Androgens in Peri- and Postmenopausal Women

The ovaries produce significant amounts of androgen during and after the childbearing years. Testosterone increases sex drive in both men and women.

**Table 8–6.**    Common doses and preparations of estrogen and progestin

| Formulation | Dose (mg) |
|---|---|
| Estrogen preparations | |
|   Conjugated equine estrogen | 0.3, 0.625, 1.25 |
|   Piperazine estrone sulfate | 0.6, 1.2 |
|   Micronized estradiol | 1, 2 |
|   Conjugated estrogen vaginal cream | 1.25, 2.5 |
|   Transdermal estradiol patch | 0.025, 0.0375, 0.05, 0.06, 0.075, 0.1 |
|   Estradiol vaginal ring | 0.05, 0.1 |
| Progestin preparations | |
|   Medroxyprogesterone acetate | 2.5, 5, 10 |
|   Megestrol acetate | 20, 40 |
|   Norethindrone | 0.35, 5 |
|   Norethindrone acetate | 5 |
|   Norgestrel | 0.075 |
|   Micronized progesterone | 100 |

Testosterone supplementation has therefore been suggested as a treatment to restore diminished or absent libido in peri- or postmenopausal women who complain of impaired sexual desire that is not attributable to psychological or physical problems, medication side effects, or relationship difficulties. A number of studies have suggested that testosterone is a useful adjunct to estrogen in the treatment of diminished libido in both naturally and surgically menopausal women (Sarrel 2000). An increase in serum SHBG secondary to estrogen replacement has been correlated with a reduction of free (active) testosterone in menopausal women (Sarrel et al. 1998). The addition of methyltestosterone significantly improved sexual sensation and desire after 8 weeks of treatment. Typical oral doses of methyltestosterone, taken in addition to standard hormone replacement, range from 1.25 mg three times per week to 2.5 mg once daily. Potential side effects of methyltestosterone include oily skin, acne, and hirsutism. Because methyltestosterone may be hepatotoxic, hepatic enzymes should be monitored at baseline and over time in women who receive this treatment. In addition, methyltestosterone may adversely affect serum cholesterol, low-density lipoprotein, and high-density lipoprotein

(HDL) profiles. Thus, women with arteriosclerosis and heart disease are not candidates for androgen treatment.

Dehydroepiandrosterone (DHEA) is a naturally occurring corticosteroid hormone that has been purported to produce wide-ranging beneficial effects and has become a popular over-the-counter treatment for the enhancement of quality of life. DHEA has been reported to diminish fat, enhance muscle mass, boost libido, improve depression, increase feelings of well-being, and prevent a variety of illnesses (heart disease, cancer, diabetes, Parkinson's disease, and Alzheimer's disease) (Skolnick 1996). Because many of the claims regarding the beneficial effects of DHEA relate to the reversal of age-related conditions, it has been suggested that DHEA may be useful in treating menopausal symptoms. The results of the first double-blind, placebo-controlled trial of DHEA for the treatment of major depression revealed a statistically significant antidepressant effect (Wolkowitz et al. 1999). Despite the large numbers of reports in the medicine and psychiatry literature that suggest that DHEA may eventually have a wide variety of therapeutic applications, its efficacy and long-term safety require further study. Known short-term side effects of DHEA include acne, hirsutism, deepening of the voice, amenorrhea, nasal congestion, and headache. Other concerns related to DHEA that have been raised include decreased HDL cholesterol levels in women, cardiac arrhythmias, and possible tumorigenic effects. Until more is known about both the beneficial effects and possible adverse effects of DHEA, it is prudent to discourage patients from using this agent.

# Evaluation and Treatment of Depression

The psychiatric evaluation of the middle-aged depressed woman should include an assessment of menstrual cycle patterns, vasomotor symptoms, and sexual function. Because a woman may not be aware of vasomotor symptoms occurring at night, it is important to ask whether her nightclothes or sheets are damp or wet when she wakes up. Sleep disruption in middle-aged women is often the result of nighttime hot flashes and night sweats.

Hormonal evaluation on day 2 or 3 of the menstrual cycle may reveal elevated FSH and depressed estradiol levels. Thyroid function should also be evaluated, because women over age 40 years are at particular risk for thyroid disorders, and hypothyroidism may contribute to depressive symptoms. The patient should be referred for a full medical examination to rule out health problems (e.g., autoimmune disorders, endocrine disorders, heart disease, cancer) that may contribute to depressed mood.

Treatment of the perimenopausal woman who meets the criteria for a major depressive episode involves the usual psychiatric treatment modalities, including psychotherapy and pharmacotherapy. Study findings lend support to the use of selective serotonin reuptake inhibitors or a selective norepinephrine reuptake inhibitor antidepressant (venlafaxine) to treat both vasomotor and depressive symptoms. In a randomized, double-blind, placebo-controlled study, paroxetine reduced the frequency of postmenopausal hot flashes by about 60% (Stearns et al. 2003). Preliminary reports have suggested that fluoxetine and venlafaxine improve hot flashes in breast cancer patients (Loprinzi et al. 1998; Loprinzi et al. 1999). Although preliminary data for the use of estrogen to treat major and minor perimenopausal depression are encouraging (Cohen et al. 2003; Schmidt et al. 2000; Soares et al. 2001), larger studies are needed before estrogen can be recommended as a primary modality to treat these conditions, particularly in view of the concerns regarding risks as defined by the WHI. Early data do not support the short-term use of estrogen for the treatment of depression in postmenopausal women (Cohen et al. 2003; Morrison et al. 2004).

As noted earlier, short-term hormone therapy is approved for the treatment of disruptive vasomotor symptoms and urogenital atrophy and for the prevention of osteoporosis. If a perimenopausal woman is experiencing mild to moderate depressed mood, irritability, insomnia, and poor concentration in association with frequent or distressing hot flashes or night sweats, a trial of hormone therapy will relieve vasomotor symptoms and may also improve psychological symptoms.

Because depressive symptoms in the perimenopausal years may be associated with psychosocial stressors, these stressors should be addressed in the treatment. The perimenopausal woman should be encouraged to discuss other sources of stress, including possible interpersonal stress, changing sexuality on her part or that of her partner, new-onset health problems, shifting role expectations, and new responsibilities, such as caring for aging and ill parents. In addition to individual psychotherapy, important aspects of treatment include referrals to caregiver support groups, assistance with obtaining financial support, and attention to chronic medical problems.

## Menopause, Hormone Therapy, and Cognition

As women pass through the menopausal transition, they frequently complain about memory loss and poor concentration. These complaints are generally mild and may be related to sleep deprivation secondary to perimenopausal vasomotor symptoms. Postmenopausal women also may experience a reduction in cognitive functioning. Mild decreases in cognition that are not indicative of severe dementia occur in at least 10% of persons older than age 65 years. In addition, postmenopausal women appear to be at increased risk for Alzheimer's disease, compared to men of similar age (Morrison and Tweedy 2000).

Estrogen has been shown in animals to have brain-enhancing effects, including stimulation of neuronal regeneration, activation of neurotropic growth factors, improvement of carotid artery blood flow, and promotion of cholinergic neuron growth (Barrett-Conner and Kritz-Silverstein 1993; Tang et al. 1996). Despite these intriguing animal data, data in humans have been mixed. A meta-analysis of epidemiological studies showed that estrogen therapy improved cognitive performance in recently menopausal women with vasomotor symptoms but not in asymptomatic menopausal women (Yaffe et al. 1998). Further, in a multicenter clinical trial of older women with mild to moderate Alzheimer's disease, estrogen did not appear to arrest the progression of cognitive decline over 1 year of treatment (Mulnard et al. 2000). Although observational studies indicate approximately a 30% decreased risk for the development of dementia among women receiving estrogen replacement, these data are confounded by the demographic characteristics of women who choose to take estrogen. For example, women who receive hormone therapy are more likely to be in good health and to be well educated than are women who do not take hormones, and these factors are associated with a reduced risk of dementia (Yaffe et al. 1998). As noted earlier, results of the WHIMS indicate that hormone treatment increases the risk for dementia in postmenopausal women (Shumaker et al. 2003; Shumaker et al. 2004)

## Summary

The short-term use of estrogen therapy for the treatment of intolerable vasomotor symptoms and urogenital atrophy continues to be acceptable. In peri- and postmenopausal women who are at high risk for osteoporosis, estrogen therapy may also be appropriate. What has become increasingly clear is that the widespread use of hormone therapy—either as estrogen monotherapy or in an estrogen/progestin combination—to prevent coronary heart disease and cognitive decline in postmenopausal women is not warranted, despite the numerous observational studies that had suggested otherwise. It remains to be seen whether short-term (e.g., 1–2 years) use of estrogen is a viable treatment option for depression in perimenopausal women.

# References

American Psychiatric Association: Diagnostic and Statistical Manual: Mental Disorders. Washington, DC, American Psychiatric Association, 1952

American Psychiatric Association: Diagnostic and Statistical Manual of Mental Disorders, 2nd Edition. Washington, DC, American Psychiatric Association, 1968

American Psychiatric Association: Diagnostic and Statistical Manual of Mental Disorders, 3rd Edition. Washington, DC, American Psychiatric Association, 1980

Amsterdam J, Garcia-Espana F, Fawcett J, et al: Fluoxetine efficacy in menopausal women with and without estrogen replacement. J Affect Disord 55:11–17, 1999

Anderson GL, Limacher M, Assaf AR, et al: Effects of conjugated equine estrogen in postmenopausal women with hysterectomy: the Women's Health Initiative randomized controlled trial. JAMA 291:1701–1712, 2004

Avis NE, McKinlay SM: A longitudinal analysis of women's attitudes toward the menopause: results from the Massachusetts Women's Health Study. Maturitas 13:65–79, 1991

Avis NE, McKinlay SM: The Massachusetts Women's Health Study: an epidemiologic investigation of the menopause. J Am Med Womens Assoc 50:45–49, 1995

Barrett-Connor E, Kritz-Silverstein D: Estrogen replacement therapy and cognitive function in older women. JAMA 269:2637–2641, 1993

Bromberger JT, Meyer PM, Kravitz HM, et al: Psychologic distress and natural menopause: a multiethnic community study. Am J Public Health 91:1435–1442, 2001

Cohen LS, Soares CN, Poitras JR, et al: Short-term use of estradiol for depression in perimenopausal and postmenopausal women: a preliminary report. Am J Psychiatry 160:1519–1522, 2003

Dennerstein L, Dudley E, Burger H: Are changes in sexual functioning during midlife due to aging or menopause? Fertil Steril 76:456-460, 2001

Espeland MA, Rapp SA, Shumaker SA, et al: Conjugated equine estrogens and global cognitive function in postmenopausal women: Women's Health Initiative Memory Study. JAMA 291:2959–2968, 2004

Freeman EW, Sammel MD, Liu L, et al: Hormones and menopausal status as predictors of depression in women in transition to menopause. Arch Gen Psychiatry 61:62–70, 2004

Gelfand MM: Sexuality among older women. J Womens Health Gend Based Med 9 (suppl 1):S15–S20, 2000

Grady D: Postmenopausal hormones—therapy for symptoms only. New Engl J Med 348:1835–1837, 2003

Grady D, Rubin SM, Petitti DB, et al: Hormone therapy to prevent disease and prolong life in postmenopausal women. Ann Intern Med 117:1016–1037, 1992

Hillard PJA: Gynecologic disorders and surgery, in Psychological Aspects of Women's Health Care. Edited by Stewart DE, Stotland NL. Washington, DC, American Psychiatric Press, 1993, pp 267–289

Kaufert PA, Gilbert P, Tate R: The Manitoba Project: a reexamination of the link between menopause and depression. Maturitas 14:143–155, 1992

Khastgir G, Studd JW, Catalan J: The psychological outcome of hysterectomy. Gynecol Endocrinol 14:132–141, 2000

Loprinzi CL, Pisansky TM, Fonseca R, et al: Pilot evaluation of venlafaxine hydrochloride for the therapy of hot flashes in cancer survivors. J Clin Oncology 16:2377–2381, 1998

Loprinzi CL, Quella SK, Sloan JA, et al: Preliminary data from a randomized evaluation of fluoxetine (Prozac) for treating hot flashes in breast cancer survivors (abstract). Breast Cancer Res Treat 57:34, 1999

Maartens LW, Knottnerus JA, Pop VJ: Menopausal transition and increased depressive symptomatology: a community based prospective study. Maturitas 42:195–200, 2002

Maas CP, Weijenborg PT, ter Kuile MM: The effect of hysterectomy on sexual functioning. Annu Rev Sex Res 14:83–113, 2003

Morrison MF, Tweedy K: Effects of estrogen on mood and cognition in aging women. Psychiatr Ann 30:113–119, 2000

Morrison MF, Kallan MJ, Ten Have T, et al: Lack of efficacy of estradiol for depression in postmenopausal women: a randomized, controlled trial. Biol Psychiatry 55:406–412, 2004

Mulnard RA, Cotman CW, Kawas C, et al: Estrogen replacement therapy for treatment of mild to moderate Alzheimer disease: a randomized controlled trial. JAMA 283:1007–1015, 2000

Rapp SR, Espeland MA, Shumaker SA, et al: Effect of estrogen plus progestin on global cognitive function in postmenopausal women: the Women's Health Initiative Memory Study: a randomized controlled trial. JAMA 289:2663–2672, 2003

Rhodes JC, Kjerulff KH, Langenberg PW, et al: Hysterectomy and sexual functioning. JAMA 282:1934–1941, 1999

Roovers JP, van der Bom JG, van der Vaart CH, et al: Hysterectomy and sexual well-being: prospective observational study of vaginal hysterectomy, subtotal abdominal hysterectomy, and total hysterectomy. BMJ 327:774–778, 2003

Rossouw JE, Anderson GL, Prentice RL, et al: Risks and benefits of estrogen plus progestin in healthy postmenopausal women: principal results from the Women's Health Initiative randomized controlled trial. JAMA 288:321–333, 2002

Sarrel PM: Effects of hormone replacement therapy on sexual psychophysiology and behavior in postmenopause. J Womens Health Gend Based Med 9 (suppl 1):S25–S32, 2000

Sarrel P, Dobay B, Wiita B: Estrogen and estrogen-androgen replacement in postmenopausal women dissatisfied with estrogen-only therapy: sexual behavior and neuroendocrine responses. J Reprod Med 43:847–856, 1998

Schmidt PJ, Nieman L, Danaceau MA, et al: Estrogen replacement in perimenopause-related depression: a preliminary report. Am J Obstet Gynecol 183:414–420, 2000

Schneider LS, Small GW, Hamilton SH, et al: Estrogen replacement and response to fluoxetine in a multicenter geriatric depression trial. Am J Geriatr Psychiatry 5:97–106, 1997

Shifren JL, Schiff I: The aging ovary. J Womens Health Gend Based Med 9 (suppl 1): S3–S7, 2000

Shumaker SA, Legault C, Rapp SR, et al: Estrogen plus progestin and the incidence of dementia and mild cognitive impairment in postmenopausal women: the Women's Health Initiative Memory Study: a randomized controlled trial. JAMA 289:2651–2662, 2003

Shumaker SA, Legault C, Kuller L, et al: Conjugated equine estrogens and incidence of probable dementia and mild cognitive impairment in postmenopausal women: Women's Health Initiative Memory Study. JAMA 291:2947–2958, 2004

Skolnick AA: Scientific verdict still out on DHEA. JAMA 276:1365–1367, 1996

Soares CN, Almeida OP, Joffe H, et al: Efficacy of estradiol for the treatment of depressive disorders in perimenopausal women: a double-blind, randomized, placebo-controlled trial. Arch Gen Psychiatry 58:529–534, 2001

Stearns V, Beebe KL, Iyengar M, et al: Paroxetine controlled release in the treatment of menopausal hot flashes: a randomized controlled trial. JAMA 289:2827–2834, 2003

Stone AB, Pearlstein TB: Evaluation and treatment of changes in mood, sleep and sexual functioning associated with menopause. Obstet Gynecol Clin North Am 21:391–403, 1994

Tang MX, Jacobs D, Stern Y, et al: Effect of oestrogen during menopause on risk and age at onset of Alzheimer's disease. Lancet 348:429–432, 1996

Weiss G, Skurnick JH, Goldsmith LT, et al: Menopause and hypothalamic-pituitary sensitivity to estrogen. JAMA 292:2991–2996, 2004; erratum in JAMA 293:163, 2005

Wolkowitz OM, Reus VI, Keebler A, et al: Double-blind treatment of major depression with dehydroepiandrosterone. Am J Psychiatry 156:646–649, 1999

Yaffe K, Sawaya G, Lieberburg I, et al: Estrogen therapy in postmenopausal women: effects on cognitive function and dementia. JAMA 279:688–695, 1998

# 9

# Gender Issues in the Treatment of Mental Illness

## Schizophrenia in Women

### Epidemiology

Significant gender differences exist in the course and manifestation of schizophrenia. Although the incidence of schizophrenia has been widely reported to be approximately equal in men and women, a recent meta-analysis of the literature from the past two decades reported that the incidence risk ratio for men relative to women is between 1.31 and 1.42 (Aleman et al. 2003). The authors of this study suggested that these findings may reflect an increasing preponderance of schizophrenia in men in recent years. This increase may be related to the use of illicit drugs, which may precipitate the illness in genetically vulnerable men. Because oral contraceptives contain estrogen, which has dopamine-blocking effects in animal studies, the use of these agents may have had a protective effect in some women.

In men, rates of new-onset schizophrenia reach a peak between ages 15 and 24 years. For women, the peak occurs between ages 20 and 29 years. About 15% of women with schizophrenia do not develop the illness until their mid- or late 40s, possibly reflecting a response to the perimenopausal decline of estrogen (Aleman et al. 2003) (Table 9–1). For men, onset of the illness after age 40 years is rare. The diagnosis of schizophrenia is more likely to be delayed in women, in some cases possibly because of misdiagnosis of either

**Table 9–1.**    Gender differences in schizophrenia

*Compared with men, women...*

Are less likely to have structural brain abnormalities.

Tend to receive the diagnosis later.

Are more likely to have relatives with the illness.

Are more likely to have late-onset schizophrenia.

Are less likely to abuse substances.

Are less likely to commit suicide.

Tend to exhibit more positive and fewer negative symptoms.

Tend to exhibit more affective symptoms.

Tend to respond to lower doses of neuroleptics premenopausally.

Maintain better social functioning (e.g., higher rate of employment, marriage).

major depression or bipolar disorder, as schizophrenia in women tends to be more affect-laden (Seeman 2004).

Other gender differences include a more favorable premorbid history in women and more favorable outcome, at least in the first 15 years after onset of the illness (Grigoriadis and Seeman 2002; Seeman 2004). Women with schizophrenia tend to experience more affective and positive symptoms and fewer negative symptoms (e.g., social withdrawal and lack of drive) than men. In addition, women who present initially with schizophrenia after age 45 years typically suffer fewer negative symptoms than either men of the same age with schizophrenia or age-matched women with early-onset schizophrenia (Lindamer et al. 1999). Structural brain abnormalities, such as increased ventricle size and decreased hippocampal volume, appear to be less common in women with schizophrenia than in men with the disorder (Cowell et al. 1996). Because relatives of women with schizophrenia are more likely to develop the illness, compared with relatives of men with schizophrenia, some researchers have suggested that schizophrenia is a more heritable illness in women and that environmental factors, such as birth complications, may be of more etiological significance in men (Castle and Murray 1991).

## Special Considerations in Treatment

Issues in the treatment of women with schizophrenia are listed in Table 9–2. Some, but not all studies suggest that, compared with men, women respond better to treatment and may require lower doses of medication before menopause (Seeman 2004). Findings of a more favorable treatment response and course of illness in women have supported the speculation that estrogen may have a protective effect against schizophrenia (Szymanski et al. 1995). It is noteworthy that symptomatic exacerbation of schizophrenia and an increase in psychiatric hospital admission rates have been observed during the low-estrogen phases of the menstrual cycle (Bergemann et al. 2002; Choi et al. 2001; Seeman 1996; Szymanski et al. 1995) and in perimenopausal and postmenopausal years (Seeman 1986).

**Table 9–2.** Special issues in treating women with schizophrenia

Assess for possible symptomatic variation across the menstrual cycle and perimenopausally.

Inquire about menstrual irregularities, amenorrhea, galactorrhea; measure serum prolactin levels.

Counsel about avoiding unwanted sexual advances.

Counsel about birth control.

Inquire about recent unprotected intercourse; consider obtaining pregnancy test.

The menstrual patterns of women with schizophrenia should be monitored routinely. Careful clinical monitoring of symptoms in relation to the menstrual cycle, perhaps with the use of a diary, may be useful. If such monitoring indicates premenstrual worsening of symptoms, exacerbation of symptoms may be minimized by raising antipsychotic doses during the symptomatic premenstrual days. Women with schizophrenia should also be monitored carefully for worsening illness as they transition into menopause, as it may be necessary to increase antipsychotic doses at this time.

In a small double-blind, placebo-controlled study of acutely symptomatic premenopausal antipsychotic-treated women with schizophrenia, the use of transdermal estradiol as an adjunctive treatment resulted in significant improvement in psychotic symptoms (Kulkarni et al. 2001). Further studies are needed to determine whether estrogen may have a role as an adjunctive agent for the treatment of women with schizophrenia. Estrogen therapy in postmenopausal women has been associated with increased risks for cardiac events, pulmonary embolism, stroke, dementia, and breast cancer (Rossouw et al. 2002), and therefore estrogen therapy should not be used for the treatment of psychiatric symptoms unless its benefits clearly outweigh its risks. Certain antipsychotic medications (e.g., risperidone, haloperidol, fluphenazine) can cause irregularities in the menstrual cycle by increasing levels of the pituitary hormone prolactin, which in turn inhibits release of folliclestimulating hormone (FSH) from the pituitary. As FSH is necessary for maturation of the ovarian follicles, a hyperprolactinemic state can prevent ovulation. Furthermore, hyperprolactinemia and the ensuing hypoestrogenemia can lead to a reduction in bone mineral density (Seeman 2004). Amenorrhea (i.e., absence of the menstrual cycle) is not unusual when prolactin levels exceed 60 ng/mL (normal prolactin levels are 5–25 ng/mL) (Seeman 1983). Galactorrhea, or nipple discharge, may also occur with elevated prolactin levels. If prolactin levels exceed 100 ng/mL, a brain-imaging study (preferably magnetic resonance imaging [MRI]), should be performed to rule out a prolactin-secreting pituitary tumor. Additional causes of elevated prolactin include pregnancy, nursing, stress, weight loss, opiate use, and use of oral contraceptives (Marken et al. 1992). For women of childbearing age with menstrual cycle disturbances, β-human chorionic gonadotropin (β-HCG) levels should be measured to test for pregnancy. Other relatively common causes of irregularities in the menstrual cycle include hypothyroidism and primary hyperprolactinemia. If hyperprolactinemia is determined to be secondary to the use of an antipsychotic agent, the dose should be reduced or the medication should be replaced with one of the newer antipsychotic agents, such as olanzapine, ziprasidone, aripiprazole, or quetiapine, which do not tend to raise prolactin levels. As an alternative, dopamine agonists such as bromocriptine (2.5–7.5 mg bid) or cabergoline (0.5 mg/week) can be used to reduce prolactin levels. At these low doses, bromocriptine does not appear to exacerbate psychosis. The effect of cabergoline on psychotic symptoms has not been evaluated. Cabergoline requires only once or twice weekly dosing and produces few side effects, whereas bromocriptine must be taken daily and can cause significant nausea. To minimize the nausea, bromocriptine should be taken with food. A third strategy is initiation of an oral contraceptive. This approach returns the patient to regular menstrual cycling and, by restoring estrogen, protects against the long-term adverse effects of a hypoestrogenic state, such as osteoporosis. In addition, this approach has the advantage of providing contraception. Prolactin levels, however, may rise with use of oral contraceptives and thus should be monitored closely. If prolactin levels rise or amenorrhea persists, the woman should be referred for a gynecological and endocrinological evaluation.

Women with schizophrenia are at particular risk for pregnancy resulting from ineffective use of birth control and high rates of sexual assault. Even women with antipsychotic-induced amenorrhea may occasionally ovulate and thus can become pregnant. Teaching women with schizophrenia about methods for birth control and strategies for avoiding unwanted sexual advances is an important aspect of treatment. Women with schizophrenia who become pregnant are at increased risk for stillbirth, preterm delivery, and low-birth-weight babies, and their newborns are at increased risk for sudden infant death syndrome (Bennedsen et al. 2001; Nilsson et al. 2002; Jablonsky et al. 2005). Women with schizophrenia are also at increased risk for giving birth to an infant with cardiovascular congenital anomalies (Jablonsky et al. 2005). Although the reasons for these findings are not clear, research in obstetric clinics has found that pregnant women with schizophrenia typically attend fewer than 50% of prenatal care appointments (Kelly et al. 1999), and inadequate prenatal care significantly increases the relative risk of preterm birth and postnatal death (Vintzileos et al. 2002a, 2002b). Clinicians working with pregnant schizophrenia patients should strongly encourage them to obtain regular prenatal care in an effort to improve their birth outcomes.

# Mood Disorders in Women

## Depression

### *Epidemiology*

A number of large epidemiological studies have consistently found that women are more likely than men to experience depressive disorders (Choi et al. 2001; Weissman et al. 1984, 1991). The Epidemiologic Catchment Area study, the largest survey of psychiatric disorders in North America, reported a female-to-male ratio of 1.96:1 for major depression, with a lifetime prevalence of mood disorders of 10.2% in women and 5.2% in men (Weissman et al. 1991). Researchers in the National Comorbidity Survey used a structured psychiatric interview to evaluate a representative sample of the general population and reported higher rates of depression in both sexes (Table 9–3), with a lifetime rate of major depression of 21.3% in women and 12.7% in men, producing a female-to-male ratio of 1.68:1 (Kessler et al. 1993, 1994). The increased prevalence of depression in women begins in adolescence and is a cross-cultural phenomenon (Bland et al. 1988; Wells et al. 1989; Wittchen et al. 1992). Although most exogenous stressors influence the risk for depression similarly in both women and men, women appear to be more likely to become depressed in response to interpersonal difficulties within their close family networks, and men appear more likely to become depressed in response to occupational difficulties (job loss, work problems) (Kendler et al. 2001). Although the female preponderance for depression has been shown across countries (Wittchen et al. 1992), it does not necessarily occur in select populations within these countries. Thus, although Jewish individuals have higher rates of depression than do other population groups, the female-to-male ratio for depression is 1:1; the lack of gender difference may be due to the lower rate of alcoholism among Jewish men and the inverse relationship between alcoholism and major depression (Levav et al. 1997). However, for dysthymia, the prevalence is twice as high in women, with lifetime rates of 5.4% for women and 2.6% for men (Kessler et al. 1993). The preponderance of depression in women is even higher for atypical depression (i.e., depression characterized by mood reactivity and at least one of the following symptoms: hypersomnia, hyperphagia, leaden paralysis, rejection sensitivity) and for seasonal affective disorder (SAD) (Rosenthal et al. 1984). Although female gender increases the risk for major depression and dysthymia, data from the National Comorbidity Survey suggest that a prior history of an anxiety disorder increases the risk for these conditions still more (Parker and Hadzi-Pavlovic 2001) These findings suggest that the female preponderance for depression and dysthymia might be determined primarily by a gender difference in the prevalence of anxiety disorders (Parker and Hadzi-Pavlovic 2001).

### Special Considerations in Treatment

Whether there are gender-based differences in response rates for different antidepressants is a subject of controversy. Thus, although some authors have suggested that, compared with men, women respond better to selective serotonin reuptake inhibitors than to the tricyclic antidepressant imipramine (Kornstein et al. 2000), data from more than 1,700 depressed men and women indicate that for adult patients up to age 65 years, response rates are equivalent for both tricyclic antidepressants and fluoxetine (Quitkin et al.

**Table 9–3.**  National Comorbidity Survey rates of affective disorders in men and women

| Affective disorder | Men (%) | | Women (%) | | Total (%) | |
|---|---|---|---|---|---|---|
| | Lifetime | 12 months | Lifetime | 12 months | Lifetime | 12 months |
| Major depressive episode | 12.7 | 7.7 | 21.3 | 12.9 | 17.1 | 10.3 |
| Manic episode | 1.6 | 1.4 | 1.7 | 1.3 | 1.6 | 1.3 |
| Dysthymia | 4.8 | 2.1 | 8.0 | 3.0 | 6.4 | 2.5 |
| Any affective disorder | 14.7 | 8.5 | 23.9 | 14.1 | 19.3 | 11.3 |

*Source.*  Data extracted from Kessler et al. 1994.

2002). Women seemed to have a statistically superior response to monoamine oxidase inhibitor antidepressants, but that difference did not appear to be clinically significant (Quitkin et al. 2002). A recent study found that response to tricyclic antidepressants did not vary by gender (Wohlfarth et al. 2004). In providing pharmacological treatment to women of reproductive age, it is important to keep in mind the possibility of pregnancy. Therefore, sexually active women should be advised to use an effective method of contraception. For women who are planning to conceive and who may require continued use of medication during pregnancy, choosing an antidepressant that appears safe during pregnancy may prevent the need to switch medications after conception. Some women with depression experience premenstrual exacerbation of their symptoms (Wohlfarth et al. 2004) and thus may experience a worsening of premenstrual symptoms despite successful treatment of depression at other times of the month (see Chapter 2, section titled "Evaluation"). For women who exhibit monthly exacerbation of a depression that is otherwise responsive to pharmacotherapy, it may be useful to chart the timing of the symptoms. If there appears to be a consistent premenstrual exacerbation of depression, an increase in antidepressant dose 7–10 days before the onset of menses may help maintain euthymia throughout the cycle (Jensvold et al. 1992; Yonkers 1997).

Certain antidepressants (including tricyclic antidepressants and selective serotonin reuptake inhibitors) may cause hyperprolactinemia as a result of their serotonergic activity (Marken et al. 1992). Although this effect is relatively rare, it is important to keep it in mind, particularly for patients taking antidepressants who complain of amenorrhea, galactorrhea (nipple discharge), or breast pain.

Women are far more likely than men to experience an eating disorder, and many women with eating disorders have comorbid depression. Because patients with anorexia or bulimia may have electrolyte imbalances that put them at particular risk for seizures, medications that reduce the seizure threshold (bupropion, clomipramine, maprotiline) should be avoided.

Women are at increased risk for depression during approximately the first 4–8 weeks after delivery (see Chapter 5, section titled "Postpartum Depression"), and this increase in risk is particularly true for women with a history of depression. For some women, prophylaxis with an antidepressant, begun 1–2 days after delivery, may decrease the likelihood of an episode of postpartum-onset major depression (Wisner and Wheeler 1994). Some data show that women with a history of depression related to the use of oral contraceptives or to the premenstruum or postpartum period are at risk of perimenopausal depression (Freeman et al. 2004; Stewart and Boydell 1993). Particularly in women with histories of depression, longitudinal monitoring for recurrence of depression at vulnerable points in the reproductive life cycle may allow for the rapid implementation of treatment and the prevention of a relapse.

## Bipolar Disorder

### Epidemiology

Although bipolar disorder occurs equally frequently in men and women, there are significant gender differences in its course and manifestation (Table 9–4). It has generally been accepted that women with the disorder appear to experience more depressive episodes than do men with the disorder, whereas men experience more manic episodes (Leibenluft 1996). However, two studies, one retrospective and one prospective, suggested that there may not be significant gender differences in the total number of depressive or manic episodes (Hendrick et al. 2000; Winokur et al. 1994). Dysphoric (mixed) mania may be more common in women (Leibenluft 1996). Women with bipolar disorder are approximately two times as likely as men with the disorder to experience rapid cycling, defined as four or more affective episodes per year (Tondo and Baldessarini 1998). The number of cycles occurring in men and women with rapid cycling does not appear to be significantly different, and both men and women appear to respond similarly to lithium treatment (Tondo and Baldessarini 1998). Why rapid-cycling bipolar disorder should occur more often in women is unclear. It may result from women's greater likelihood of being treated with antidepressants, which may precipitate rapid cycling (Wehr and Goodwin 1979). In addition, thyroid dysfunction is more common in women, and hypothyroidism has been implicated in rapid cycling. The data on the relationship between thyroid function and rapid cycling are mixed, as are the data on the use of thyroid supplementation for treatment of rapid cycling. Although more men than women with bipolar disorder experience comorbid alcohol and substance use disorders, when women and men with bipolar disorder were compared to women and men in the general population, the relative risk of comorbid alcohol and substance use disorders was greater for women with bipolar disorder (Frye et al. 2003).

**Table 9–4.**    Gender differences in bipolar disorder

*Compared with men, women...*

Are more likely to have rapid cycling.

Are more likely to develop lithium-induced hypothyroidism.

Experience more depressions.

May experience more dysphoric manias.

Are at increased risk for alcoholism, compared to the general population.

Women with bipolar disorder may experience premenstrual relapse or exacerbation of symptoms (Hendrick et al. 1996). Mood fluctuations in women with rapid-cycling bipolar disorder, however, do not appear to vary consistently with the menstrual cycle (Leibenluft 1996; Leibenluft et al. 1999). Daily charting of moods allows an assessment of the relationship between menstrual cycle phases and mood changes. For women whose mood consistently deteriorates premenstrually, it is helpful to measure blood levels of medication both premenstrually and in the week postmenses, as serum levels of mood stabilizers may fluctuate across the menstrual cycle (Tondo and Baldessarini 1998).

*Special Considerations in Treatment*

Gender-specific differences in presentation, clinical course, physiology, concomitant medications, and reproductive phase of life are all factors that should be considered when choosing among treatment options for bipolar disorder in women (Burt and Rasgon 2004). Special issues in the treatment of women with bipolar disorder are listed in Table 9–5. Because women who take lithium are at significant risk of developing lithium-induced hypothyroidism, thyroid function should be monitored at least every 6 months. Women older than age 40 years are particularly at risk for thyroid dysfunction, whether it is lithium-induced or results from another etiology.

By inducing hormone clearance and metabolism, carbamazepine, oxcarbazepine, and topiramate may reduce the efficacy of oral contraceptives. Women with bipolar disorder who are taking these antiepileptic drugs and oral contraceptives should therefore be advised to use a different or an additional form of contraception. Postmenopausal women taking carbamazepine, oxcarbazepine, or topiramate may find that they need higher doses of hor-

**Table 9–5.** Special concerns in treating women with bipolar disorder

Symptoms may recur or worsen premenstrually.

Medication levels may fluctuate across the menstrual cycle.

Carbamazepine, oxcarbazepine, and topiramate may render oral contraceptives ineffective through their induction of liver enzymes.

Estrogen-containing oral contraceptives may reduce the level of lamotrigine.

Psychotropic agents (e.g., antipsychotics, valproate) may produce menstrual-cycle disturbances.

Mood-stabilizing medications, especially valproate and carbamazepine, are associated with relatively high rates of fetal anomalies when used during the first trimester of pregnancy (see Chapter 4, sections titled "Use of Psychiatric Medications During Pregnancy" and "Mood Stabilizers").

Valproate and carbamazepine may increase the risk for osteoporosis.

Women with bipolar disorder are at significant risk for postpartum psychosis (see Chapter 5, section titled "Postpartum Psychosis").

mone replacement to reduce hypoestrogenemia-induced vasomotor symptoms (hot flashes, night sweats). Because oral contraceptives can reduce lamotrigine plasma levels by up to 60%, it is prudent for women who are taking both agents to have their lamotrigine doses monitored and adjusted as needed to maintain clinical efficacy (Sabers et al. 2001).

Several studies have examined whether the use of valproate puts women at an increased risk of developing polycystic ovary syndrome (PCOS), a heterogeneous condition characterized by irregular or absent menstrual cycles, hirsutism, and insulin resistance (Isojarvi et al. 1993; McIntyre et al. 2003; Rasgon 2004; Rasgon et al. 2000). Although the pathophysiology of PCOS is not well understood, hyperinsulinemia—a potential side effect of some medications, including valproate—is believed to play a role. The available information on the association between valproate and PCOS has been inconsistent, although some studies have identified high rates of menstrual disturbances among women with bipolar disorder, regardless of which medication they take (Isojarvi et al. 1993; Rasgon et al. 2000). Until more data are available, clinicians should be watchful for symptoms of menstrual irregularities and/or PCOS in patients with bipolar disorder, especially if they are taking valproate (Luef et al. 2002). Certain antipsychotic agents (e.g., risperidone,

haloperidol) may also potentially cause amenorrhea or menstrual disturbances by elevating serum prolactin levels.

Obtaining a menstrual history is essential for assessing patterns of
bipolar-disorder symptom exacerbation in relation to the menstrual cycle and
for monitoring psychotropic-induced disturbances of the menstrual cycle
pattern.

Some studies have reported an increased risk for osteoporosis among
women taking carbamazepine or valproate (Pack and Morrell 2004). Several
mechanisms have been suggested for this finding, including an increase in the
metabolism of vitamin D, resistance to parathyroid hormone, and impaired
calcium absorption. Although not all studies have observed this risk, it is
probably wise to counsel women who take carbamazepine or valproate about
good bone health practices, including adequate intake of calcium and vitamin
D, regular weight-bearing exercise, adequate sunlight exposure, and avoidance of nicotine. Postmenopausal women who take carbamazepine or valproate should be encouraged to obtain a bone mineral density scan after
5 years of treatment.

## Seasonal Affective Disorder

### Epidemiology

Women are six times as likely as men to have seasonal affective disorder
(SAD), a condition in which depressive episodes recur in a seasonal pattern.
In "winter SAD," symptoms of depression are limited to the fall and winter
months; in "summer SAD," depression occurs in the spring and summer. For
perimenopausal women with SAD, symptoms typically occur in the fall and
winter and include subjective dysphoria, hypersomnia, severe fatigue, increased appetite, and carbohydrate craving (Levitan et al. 1998). Winter SAD
is more common in the Northern Hemisphere, whereas in the Southern
Hemisphere there is a reversed seasonal variation. For patients with recurrent
mood disorders (unipolar major depression, bipolar I disorder, or bipolar II
disorder) who experience seasonal exacerbations of depression, the seasonal
pattern specifier is added to their diagnosis. Although SAD may occur in children, the disorder tends to arise around puberty, worsen through adolescence,
and become severe around the third decade of life. The changes in mood and
behavior that characterize SAD (especially the winter type) run in families

and appear to be largely due to a biological predisposition (Madden et al. 1996). Possible etiologies implicated in SAD are circadian rhythm changes, altered melatonin secretion, or serotonin dysfunction (Levitan et al. 1998).

### Special Considerations in Treatment

Treatment of SAD includes the use of artificial light therapy (2,500 lux of light for 1–2 hours or 10,000 lux of light for 30 minutes generally administered in the morning). Although some patients respond to light administration only during the symptomatic months, maintenance light therapy may be required for patients with a more severe form of the illness. In some cases, adjunctive pharmacotherapy (generally year-round) is helpful to maintain remission from symptomatic season to season (Schwartz et al. 1996).

# Anxiety Disorders in Women

## Epidemiology

Anxiety disorders are the most prevalent psychiatric disorders, affecting one of every 10 people in the United States (Robins et al. 1984; Wells et al. 1989). As a class, anxiety disorders are more prevalent in women than in men, and women with anxiety disorders are more likely than men to experience comorbid depression (Pajer 1995; Pigott 2003). Panic with agoraphobia and generalized anxiety disorder (GAD) are two to three times more common in women than in men (Bourdon et al. 1988; Robins et al. 1984; Schneier et al. 1992), and social phobia is three to four times as common in women than in men (Schwartz et al. 1996). The rates of generalized anxiety disorder are stable in both women and men between the ages of 25 and 34 years but increase more in women older than 34 years than in age-matched men. Thus, the prevalence of GAD increases from about 1.5% in young men ages 15–24 years to 3.6% in men older than 45 years. However, in women the prevalence increases from 2.5% at age 15–24 years to 10.3% in women older than 45 years (Halbreich 2003). The rate decreases in aging men but further increases in women as they age (Robins et al. 1984). Women with panic disorder are just as likely as men to recover but are twice as likely to have a subsequent recurrence of symptoms (Yonkers et al. 1998).

Women with alcoholism are more likely to have panic disorder with agoraphobia than are men with alcoholism (Task Force on Panic Anxiety and Its

Treatments 1993). Whether agoraphobia is a precipitant for alcoholism in women is unclear. Although the prevalence rates for obsessive-compulsive disorder (OCD) are approximately equal for men and women, women appear to have a somewhat later onset than do men (average age of 25 years in women versus 20 years in men) (Flament and Rapoport 1984). Whereas the overall lifetime prevalence of exposure to traumatic events does not vary by gender (Breslau et al. 1997), lifetime rates of posttraumatic stress disorder (PTSD) are twice as high in women as in men (estimated at 10.4% for women and 5% for men) (Kessler et al. 1995). The reasons for the preponderance of anxiety disorders in women are not clear. Although genetic factors play a role in the transmission of anxiety disorders (Kendler et al. 1992, 1993), they have not been found to account for the gender differences in prevalence rates. Other possible causes for the preponderance of anxiety disorders in women include the increased prevalence rate of depression in women; the increased demands related to work and family that are currently placed on women; reproduction-related alterations in hormones; the relatively lower level of encouragement of self-sufficiency and self-confidence in girls, compared with boys; and histories of physical and sexual abuse (Pigott 2003; Zerbe 1995). With regard to PTSD, women may be culturally primed to experience traumatic events differently than men, rather than having an increased biological vulnerability. Thus, although women are more likely than men both to be molested and to subsequently develop PTSD, women are also more likely to develop PTSD after a physical assault despite the fact that men are much more likely to be victims of assault. However, although women are 10 times more likely than men to be raped, PTSD is more likely to result after this experience in men than in women (65% vs. 46%) (Yehuda 2002).

## Special Considerations in Treatment

Evaluation for anxiety should first rule out medical conditions that present with anxious symptoms. In evaluating women patients for anxiety, the clinician should give particular attention to certain medical disorders. Although it appears that women with panic disorder are more likely to experience respiration-related difficulties than men with panic disorder (Sheikh et al. 2002), complaints of chest discomfort, diaphoresis, and tachycardia warrant a thorough diagnostic evaluation for heart disease. Women with these symptoms are more likely than men to be misdiagnosed as having an anxiety disorder and less likely than men to receive a cardiac assessment (Wenger et al. 1993). Mitral valve prolapse has been associated with panic disorder and is more prevalent in women (Yonkers and Gurguis 1995). The patient's symptoms in relation to the menstrual cycle should also be evaluated, as women of reproductive age may experience premenstrual onset or worsening of anxiety. Patients with hypo- or hyperthyroidism may develop panic attacks with the onset of their thyroid condition. A thyroid panel should therefore be obtained in women reporting anxiety, tachycardia, diaphoresis, temperature intolerance, or tremor. Thyroid disease is more prevalent in women than in men, particularly in women older than age 40 years. Other medical illnesses that affect women more than men and that may present with symptoms of anxiety include systemic lupus erythematosus, iron deficiency anemia, and irritable bowel syndrome.

Nicotine and caffeine use should be assessed in women who report symptoms of anxiety and insomnia. Although in recent years the rate of cigarette smoking has declined in the general population, it has risen among teenage girls.

A full assessment of a patient's medications should be part of the workup for an anxiety disorder. A number of medications may induce symptoms of anxiety, including decongestants, steroids, herbal supplements, and appetite suppressants.

The workup should also include an assessment of past and recent traumatic events. Women are more likely than men to experience rape and sexual assault, whereas men experience higher rates of nonsexual assault. Among women, rates of PTSD after sexual and nonsexual assault are estimated at 95% and 75%, respectively, within 2 weeks of the crime. Three months after the trauma, these rates diminish to approximately 50% for sexual assault and 25% for nonsexual assault. Female victims of sexual and nonsexual assault have been successfully treated with two forms of cognitive-behavioral treatment: prolonged exposure treatment and stress inoculation training (Foa 1997). Prolonged exposure treatment involves the patient's repeated reliving of the trauma, combined with verbal recounting in therapeutic sessions, relaxation techniques, education about common reactions to trauma, and exposure to situations that remind the patient of the trauma. Stress inoculation training helps patients develop coping skills to deal with anxiety. These skills include muscle relaxation, breathing control, role-playing, thought-stopping, and self-dialogue.

Perimenopausal women may experience heat sensations, sweating, shortness of breath, and anxiety. For these women, vasomotor symptoms may be mistaken for panic or anxiety attacks (see Chapter 8, section titled "Physical changes"). A history of menstrual cycle alterations, measurement of the FSH level, and measurement of the estradiol level on day 2 or day 3 of the menstrual cycle (for women who are still cycling) can identify perimenopausal status. Hormone therapy rather than anxiolytic or antidepressant medication may suffice to resolve these symptoms if they are of vasomotor origin. Since estrogen and progestin therapy in postmenopausal women has been associated with increased risks for cardiac events, pulmonary embolism, stroke, dementia, and breast cancer, hormone therapy should be prescribed at the lowest effective dose for no more than 4–5 years (Rossouw et al. 2002).

Although women and men appear to have an equal prevalence of OCD, women seem to have more obsessions related to food and weight than do men, and women are also more likely to have comorbid anorexia (Kasvikis et al. 1986). It is therefore important to carefully evaluate all women with OCD for symptoms of restrictive-eating disorders.

# Alcohol and Substance Abuse in Women

## Alcoholism

### Epidemiology

Women are significantly less likely than men to have a drinking problem. The prevalence rate of alcoholism in men has been estimated at more than twice that in women (Walker et al. 2003). Nevertheless, alcoholism in adult women is not uncommon; its prevalence is estimated to be 6% and to be rising (Greenfield et al. 2003; Walker et al. 2003). Rates of alcoholism in young women, whose drinking patterns are approaching those of men, appear to be even higher (Walker et al. 2003).

Gender-specific physiological differences cause women to become more intoxicated than men when they drink an equal amount of alcohol per unit of body weight. Some reports suggest that alcohol dehydrogenase, the enzyme that degrades alcohol, is significantly less active in women (Blume 1994). In addition, as women have more body fat and less body water than do men, they reach higher blood alcohol levels because alcohol is diluted in total body water. Thus, although heavy drinking is considered to consist of more than four drinks a day in men, as little as one and one-half drinks a day may constitute heavy drinking for women (Cyr and Moulton 1990). Alcohol-related medical complications (e.g., peptic ulcer, liver disease, anemia, and cerebral atrophy) develop more quickly in women, and women have higher relative mortality rates from alcoholism than do men (Greenfield et al. 2003).

### Risk Factors for Alcoholism

Risk factors in women include a personal history of sexual abuse, a family history of substance abuse, and adult antisocial personality disorder (Table 9–6). Depression is a much more significant risk factor for alcohol abuse in women than in men (Blume 1994). In fact, depression tends to precede alcoholism in women, whereas in men it tends to follow alcoholism (Blume 1994). Living with a substance-abusing partner is also a major risk factor for women and can reduce the likelihood that treatment will be successful.

**Table 9–6.**   Risk factors for alcoholism in women

History of sexual abuse
Clinical depression
Living with a substance-abusing partner
Family history of alcoholism
Antisocial personality disorder

## Drug Abuse

### Epidemiology

As with alcohol abuse, the rates of abuse of hallucinogens and opiates are higher in men than in women. Cocaine and amphetamine abuse, however, are equally prevalent in men and women. Compared with men, women are less likely to inject cocaine and more likely to smoke and sniff cocaine (Gossop et al. 1994). Women may be motivated to use stimulants for weight control purposes. Rates of prescription drug abuse are higher in women, possibly because women go to doctors more often than do men. Also, women who abuse drugs or alcohol are more likely than men to have comorbid psychiatric diagnoses and thus to receive prescription medications (e.g., sedatives).

### Risk Factors for Drug Abuse

Risk factors for drug abuse include a family history of drug abuse, adult anti-social personality disorder, depression, and involvement with a drug-dependent partner (Griffin et al. 1989).

## Screening and Treatment

Special considerations in the screening and treatment of substance-abusing women are listed in Table 9–7. Any woman who presents with complaints of depression, anxiety, insomnia, sexual dysfunction, job problems, or family and marital conflicts should be assessed for substance abuse. Of particular concern is the direct request for specific prescription medications. Women who report great preoccupation with their weight should be assessed for the use of diet pills or stimulants. Although a careful history is the most important part of the evaluation, the CAGE questionnaire (Table 9–8) is a helpful screening instrument for alcoholism (Ewing 1984). Laboratory values are not reliably useful in screening for alcoholism, but they can help confirm the diagnosis. Elevated results on liver function tests, primarily the level of γ-glutamyltransferase (GGT), and a high mean corpuscular volume (MCV) suggest a history of extensive drinking. Medical problems such as peptic ulcer, hypertension, anemia, and liver disease result from heavy alcohol consumption and should prompt investigation into drinking patterns.

**Table 9–7.**  Special issues for substance-abusing women

Comorbid depressive and anxiety disorders are common.

Premenstrual tension may exacerbate substance abuse.

The amount of alcohol that produces intoxication is lower in women than in men, even after adjustment for body weight.

Medical consequences of alcoholism progress faster in women than in men.

Child care concerns may prevent a woman from obtaining treatment.

Stigmatization by society may inhibit a woman from admitting her alcohol or drug abuse.

Excessive preoccupation with weight control may lead to stimulant abuse.

Noting the presence of alcohol- and drug-related legal and employment problems is helpful in making a diagnosis of substance abuse, although more

**Table 9–8.**   CAGE questionnaire

Have you ever felt you ought to Cut down on your drinking?

Have people Annoyed you by criticizing your drinking?

Have you ever felt bad or Guilty about your drinking?

Have you ever had a drink first thing in the morning to steady your nerves or get rid of a hangover (Eye-opener)?

*Note.*   CAGE=Cut [down], Annoyed, Guilty, Eye-opener.
*Source.*   Adapted from Ewing 1984.

so in men than in women. Women who abuse alcohol or drugs, on the other hand, are more likely to have family, interpersonal, and health problems (Cyr and Moulton 1993). Because depression frequently precedes or is comorbid with substance abuse in women, all women with alcoholism or drug dependence should be assessed for current and previous depressive episodes. If a woman has a history of depression preceding her substance dependence, she is at risk for a depressive relapse as she recovers (Blume 1994; Ewing 1984; Griffin et al. 1989). Treatment of depression may reduce the likelihood that the patient will return to substance abuse. For the same reason, comorbid anxiety disorders should be treated. Addictive prescription medications are best avoided, because women with alcoholism are at risk for prescription drug abuse. An assessment for premenstrual symptoms is important, because up to two-thirds of women with alcoholism may drink to self-medicate premenstrual tension (Hendrick et al. 1996). Treatment of the premenstrual symptoms may reduce the alcohol use.

For any treatment plan to be effective, it is essential that the substance-abusing woman accept that she has an illness and recognize the interpersonal, psychological, and medical consequences of her drug use. Referrals to self-help groups—including Alcoholics Anonymous, Cocaine Anonymous, and Women for Sobriety, an all-woman support group—are important aspects of treatment. The woman's family should be involved; family support and concern may help motivate the patient to remain in recovery. Family members can benefit from referrals to Al-Anon. Because a woman's drinking or drug use pattern is greatly influenced by that of her partner, her likelihood of reaching sobriety is enhanced if her partner is sober. Thus, an evaluation of the partner's drinking or drug use patterns is important. If the partner also has a substance use problem, he or she should be encouraged to obtain treatment. Family and marital conflicts may contribute to a woman's drinking or drug use and should be explored. Attention should be given to child care needs that may interfere with a woman's ability to obtain treatment.

Societal stigmatization of women drinkers may cause women to hide drinking problems. Women may also fear losing custody of their children if they reveal their alcoholism. It is therefore essential that women with alcoholism be treated in a nonjudgmental and supportive manner. Group and individual therapy are helpful, particularly in addressing issues of shame and low self-esteem and in promoting assertiveness.

# Eating Disorders in Women

## Epidemiology and Phenomenology

The combined prevalence of anorexia nervosa and bulimia nervosa is approximately 4%, with more than 90% of cases occurring in women (Leach 1995). These illnesses typically develop in puberty and are more common in industrialized societies. Anorexia nervosa is characterized by a body weight of less than 85% of the expected weight for age and height, intense fear of gaining weight, distorted body image, and (in postmenarcheal females) amenorrhea. Anorexia nervosa is categorized as one of two types: restricting type or binge-eating/purging type. Approximately 50% of cases fall into each category (Mickley 2000). Patients with bulimia nervosa engage in episodes of binge-eating, in which they experience a sense of lack of control over eating and are excessively concerned about body image. They attempt to compensate for their food intake by self-induced vomiting; use of laxatives, diuretics, and enemas; excessive exercise; or fasting. The DSM-IV-TR diagnosis of bulimia nervosa requires that the binge-eating and compensatory behaviors occur at least twice a week for at least 3 months. The disorder is categorized as either purging type (i.e., involving the use of self-induced vomiting, laxatives, diuretics, or enemas) or nonpurging type. Patients with bulimia are usually normal in weight. Anorexia and bulimia nervosa are frequently accompanied by mood, anxiety, personality, and substance use disorders. A history of substance use disorders and a longer duration of symptoms predict worse treatment outcomes (Keel et al. 1999).

## Screening and Treatment

The evaluation of women with eating disorders should include assessments of body image; eating habits; actual and desired weight; menstrual patterns; exercise; self-induced vomiting; presence of other psychiatric disturbance; use of laxatives, diuretics, enemas, emetics, and diet pills; and abuse of alcohol and illicit substances. A number of medical complications may result from anorexia and bulimia nervosa (Table 9–9) (Becker et al. 1999). Therefore, the evaluation should include a physical and dental examination and laboratory tests for albumin, total protein, and glucose levels to help assess nutritional status. Measurement of amylase levels gives an indication of the extent of self-induced vomiting. Measurement of electrolytes, blood urea nitrogen, and creatinine levels are essential for assessing fluid and electrolyte abnormalities. A complete blood count can reveal anemia from nutritional deficiency and from internal bleeding—for example, from esophageal tears resulting from self-induced vomiting. An electrocardiogram should be obtained because cardiac conduction abnormalities may occur as a result of electrolyte imbalance, malnutrition, and ipecac-induced cardiomyopathy.

**Table 9–9.**   Medical complications of eating disorders

Cardiovascular, including electrocardiographic abnormalities (e.g., prolonged QT interval), hypotension, sinus bradycardia, atrial and ventricular arrhythmias

Gastrointestinal, including esophageal perforation, gastric rupture, rectal prolapse, elevated serum amylase

Endocrine, including metabolic alkalosis, hypokalemia, amenorrhea, osteoporosis

Orofacial, including erosion of dental enamel, parotid and submandibular gland hypertrophy

Hematological, including anemia, thrombocytopenia, leukopenia

The treatment of eating disorders should involve a multidisciplinary team including mental health professionals and a primary care physician, nutritionist, and dentist. The first priority for treatment is medical stabilization to correct malnutrition, electrolyte imbalance, and other serious medical problems. In life-threatening conditions, nasogastric tube feeding may be necessary. After medical stabilization, the treatment involves the establishment of healthful eating patterns and attention to the psychosocial precipitants of the condition (Leach 1995). Psychosocial interventions include family counseling, individual/couples psychotherapy, education, and group support. Two forms of structured, time-limited therapy have been effective in the treatment of bulimia nervosa: cognitive-behavioral therapy, which focuses on the relationship between thoughts, feelings, and behavior; and interpersonal therapy, which addresses the interpersonal stressors that precipitate disordered eating (Becker et al. 1999). Certain antidepressant medications, including fluoxetine, have been helpful for bulimia nervosa (Leach 1995). High doses (e.g., 60 mg/day) have been more effective than lower doses. Monoamine oxidase inhibitors (e.g., phenelzine, isocarboxazid) have also been effective but should be used only for patients who are able to avoid tyramine-containing foods. Antidepressant medications have been of little help in treating the symptoms of anorexia nervosa, although they are clearly indicated for associated mood and anxiety disorders. Tricyclic antidepressants can be helpful in promoting weight gain. Topiramate has been reported to be useful in reducing both bingeing and purging (Hoopes et al. 2003).

Most patients with anorexia nervosa will require intensive treatment in an inpatient setting or day program, where they can be supported in eating and weight gain restoration. Patients should be hospitalized if their body weight is 25% below normal, if they experience medical complications, or if they are refusing food. Weight gain should proceed at 2–3 lbs/week for inpatients and 1–2 lbs/week for outpatients. Patients with bulimia nervosa can usually be managed in outpatient settings. For both disorders, long-term maintenance therapy is recommended.

# Sleep Disorders in Women

In 1995, the prevalence rate of chronic insomnia was 12%, with women having a rate 1.3 times higher than that of men (Millman 1999). The risk for sleep-related difficulties rises during certain reproductive phases of women's lives: premenstrual bloating and cramping frequently disrupt sleep, as does the discomfort women experience in the third trimester of pregnancy, and night sweats produce sleep impairment in approximately one-third of perimenopausal women (Walsleben 1999).

Other common causes of insomnia include depression and anxiety disorders, side effects of medications (e.g., bronchodilators, blood pressure medications, decongestants), and use of alcohol, caffeine, nicotine, and illicit drugs. A number of medical conditions (e.g., asthma, chronic obstructive pulmonary disease, sleep apnea) produce insomnia by causing shortness of breath at night. Disruptions in circadian rhythm commonly caused by jet lag or rotating work shifts can produce insomnia. A restless limb syndrome, characterized by discomfort in the legs and sometimes in the arms, can also disrupt sleep.

A detailed history should be obtained to determine the etiology of the insomnia. If the underlying cause is a psychiatric or medical problem, the problem should be treated. The elements of sleep hygiene should be reviewed, including reduction in use of caffeine, nicotine, and alcohol; avoidance of napping during the day; maintenance of regular exercise; avoidance of excessive fluids in the evening; and maintenance of regular times for sleeping and waking up (Millman 1999). If sleep problems are associated with premenstrual phases, low-dose oral contraceptives may help, and short-term hormone therapy at the lowest effective dose will reduce night sweats that disrupt sleep in middle-aged women (Polo-Kantola et al. 1999). When sleep-promoting modalities are ineffective, it may be appropriate to prescribe a hypnotic agent. Benzodiazepines are the most common class of medications for the treatment of insomnia. A meta-analysis of controlled studies of the use of benzodiazepines for the treatment of insomnia revealed that both benzodiazepines and the nonbenzodiazepine hypnotic zolpidem produced improvement in patients with chronic insomnia (Nowell et al. 1997). However, hypnotics should be generally prescribed only for short-term use, because long-term use raises concerns of addiction and rebound insomnia after withdrawal of the medication. Sedating antidepressants (e.g., trazodone, doxepin) can be used in place of traditional agents such as benzodiazepines to treat insomnia. Few studies have evaluated the efficacy and safety of these agents to treat insomnia over the long term.

# Women Victims of Violence

## Sexual Assault

### Epidemiology

Sexual assault is defined as any form of nonconsenting sexual activity. Despite the fact that rape is a felony, most rapes are not reported (Petter and Whitehill

1998). It is estimated that only one of 10 victims of sexual assault seeks professional help (Beckman and Groetzinger 1990). Sexual assault affects women of all ages and all cultural, ethnic, and economic backgrounds. Approximately 20%–25% of all adult women, 15% of college women, and 12% of adolescent girls have experienced sexual abuse and/or assault during their lifetime, and rates are even higher for African American women (Council of Scientific Affairs, American Medical Association 1992; Silverman et al. 2001). Each year, more than 1.5 million women in the United States are physically and/or sexually abused by an intimate partner, and women are 10 times more likely than men to be killed by an intimate partner (Silverman et al. 2001). Although adolescents and young adult women are most at risk for sexual abuse by an acquaintance or someone unknown to them, older women are more likely to be sexually assaulted by marital or ex-marital partners (Council of Scientific Affairs, American Medical Association 1992).

### Special Considerations in Treatment

Most emergency departments have established protocols for rape victims that involve extensive and detailed physical evaluation, laboratory tests, and collection of evidence for possible legal action. Although both recent and past assaults threaten the psychological and physical well-being of women, only a small minority of victims actually come forth to acknowledge the assault.

Initial reactions to sexual assault vary from woman to woman and include shock, numbness, withdrawal, and denial. Physical signs often include severe tremulousness and cold sweats. The victim of assault by a stranger is often fearful of further harm, whereas the victim of assault by an acquaintance or intimate tends to be dismayed that she has been assaulted by a trusted person. When a husband or live-in partner rapes a woman, the victim may initially be numb and accepting, although she ultimately may be driven by anger and fear to seek help. It is not unusual for women who have been sexually assaulted to experience stress reactions over a period of days to weeks, including intense startle reactions, disturbed sleep and appetite, fatigue, and headache.

Virtually no victim of sexual assault escapes some form of negative psychological sequela. Initial symptoms tend to dissipate over several weeks, but symptoms often return and intensify. Over the longer term, women who have been sexually assaulted feel out of control, ashamed, vulnerable, guilty, and depressed. They often experience sexual dysfunction and aversion and may have difficulty maintaining healthy interpersonal relationships (Stewart and Robinson 1995). Symptoms of posttraumatic stress disorder are common and are particularly intense when there is a history of abuse (Stewart and Robinson 1995).

Ideally, the initial psychiatric interview should include an assessment of the patient's current symptoms, her pre-assault level of functioning, the presence of supportive significant others, and the provision of crisis management if needed for short-term safety. In fact, because the patient who has been acutely sexually assaulted is often in shock, many of the components of the initial psychiatric evaluation may be deferred. Comorbid psychiatric illness should be treated in order to facilitate management of post-rape psychiatric difficulties. It is important to educate the patient and any significant others about what she is likely to experience over the ensuing weeks. Psychotherapy is useful for assisting rape victims as they deal with new and recurring symptoms. Even if treatment is declined, the rape victim should be given the option for therapy at a later time.

Psychotherapy may use cognitive-behavioral, supportive, or psychodynamic approaches or a mixture of psychotherapeutic modalities. Group therapy is also helpful in validating the patient's experience in a safe setting where other victims can acknowledge common experiences and provide support and practical assistance. It is important for the therapist to empathically listen to the patient's recounting of her experience as it relates to her altered sense of self and as it threatens her ability to function. The therapeutic setting should provide a temporary "holding environment" until the patient is able to resurrect her own sense of security and safety (Stewart and Robinson 1995). The patient should not be pressured into revealing any details with which she is uncomfortable. Medication may be helpful in treating depression, PTSD, or general symptoms of anxiety. Although patients should be reassured that over time their stress symptoms will dissipate, they should also be advised that should symptoms recur in response to other crises or important life events a brief return to psychotherapy may be helpful.

## Domestic Violence

### Epidemiology

Women are more likely to be assaulted and injured by a current or former male partner than by all other assailants combined (Council of Scientific Affairs, American Medical Association 1992). According to a 1985 survey, physical violence aimed at a wife by her husband occurs in one of eight cohabiting couples (Council of Scientific Affairs, American Medical Association 1992). Because data on domestic violence do not fully represent the poor or the non-English-speaking population, the estimate of 2 million female victims of partner assault per year should probably be substantially increased by as much as a factor of two (Council of Scientific Affairs, American Medical Association 1992). It is noteworthy that women who have been assaulted in the past by a partner are at high risk for being assaulted again by the same partner. More than one-third of assaults involves acts of severe aggression, including choking, punching, kicking, beating, or using a weapon. Sexual assaults, psychological abuse, and threats also fall under the category of domestic violence. The rate of assaults to pregnant wives is estimated at 7% (Centers for Disease Control and Prevention 1994), and pregnant women who are abused tend to be beaten on the abdomen, in contrast to nonpregnant women, who are usually struck in the face (Stewart and Robinson 1995). At the time of the assault, women often feel that their lives are in danger, and these fears may persist after the assault. Although women do assault male and female partners, the nature of injuries to victims of domestic violence tends to be much more serious when the perpetrator is a man.

Victims of domestic violence are at risk for serious physical injury and death. Additional sequelae of domestic violence include obstetric and perinatal complications, sexually transmitted diseases, gynecologic and medical problems, depression, anxiety, eating disorders, and alcoholism (Eisenstat and Bancroft 1999). Children of battered women may suffer injury themselves and are at risk for substance abuse, suicide, school problems, violent and aggressive behavior, sleep disorders, enuresis, and chronic somatic disorders (Eisenstat and Bancroft 1999).

*Special Considerations in Treatment*

Women are often reluctant to spontaneously disclose that they have been abused by their partners. Nevertheless, because of the high prevalence of domestic violence, women who present to the offices of physicians and other health professionals with ambiguous physical findings should be evaluated in private for physical abuse. Since battering often increases during pregnancy (Eisenstat and Bancroft 1999), screening should be routinely performed during obstetric visits. Two screening questions have been found to have a sensitivity of 71% and a specificity of almost 85% in detecting domestic violence: "Do you ever feel unsafe at home?" and "Has anyone at home hit you or tried to injure you in any way?" (Eisenstat and Bancroft 1999). It is important for every health care provider to become familiar with the legal reporting requirements for domestic violence. In some states, clinicians are required to report domestic violence to local authorities. Reporting is particularly challenging, given that victims often do not wish to bring attention to the abuse because they are afraid of reprisals. Perhaps the most important function of the health care provider is to inform the patient of viable options for getting help and removing herself from danger. A national phone number, 1-800-799-SAFE, can be called for information on hospital and local community resources. Every health care provider should have a list of local resources to provide directly to women who report being abused by their partners.

Women victims of domestic violence experience acute and chronic symptoms similar to those of rape victims. During the assault, there is fear for one's life. After an assault, women tend to experience, shock, denial, isolation, confusion, psychological numbness, and fear. Over the long term, women victims of domestic violence experience sleep and appetite disturbance, startle reactions, physical complaints, fatigue, anxiety, and depression (Stewart and Robinson 1995). The fact that the abuse occurred in the context of a relationship with legal, financial, and (sometimes) shared parental relationships makes it very difficult for women to extricate themselves from the circle of abuse. Mental health clinicians should be supportive and empathic. Comorbid psychiatric conditions should be managed in order to facilitate appropriate care of the traumatic sequelae with which the patient presents. The initial therapeutic approach should be individual rather than conjoint or family, as couples' therapy is likely to precipitate defensive behaviors. The perpetrator may, however, also be willing to obtain individual therapy. If the partners wish to continue their relationship, eventually conjoint therapy should be instituted. In some cases, the use of pharmacotherapy may be needed to facilitate treatment of depression or anxiety.

# References

Aleman A, Kahn RS, Selten JP: Sex differences in the risk of schizophrenia: evidence from meta-analysis. Arch Gen Psychiatry 60:565–571, 2003

Becker AE, Grinspoon SK, Klibanski A, et al: Eating disorders. N Engl J Med 340:1092–1098, 1999

Beckman CR, Groetzinger LL: Treating sexual assault victims: a protocol for health professionals. Physician Assist 14:128–130, 1990

Bennedsen BE, Mortensen PB, Olesen A, et al: Congenital malformations, stillbirths, and infant deaths among children of women with schizophrenia. Arch Gen Psychiatry 58:674–679, 2001

Bergemann N, Parzer P, Nagl I, et al: Acute psychiatric admission and menstrual cycle phase in women with schizophrenia. Arch Womens Ment Health 5:119–126, 2002

Bland RC, Orn H, Newman SC: Lifetime prevalence of psychiatric disorders in Edmonton. Acta Psychiatr Scand Suppl 338:24–32, 1988

Blume SB: Gender differences in alcohol-related disorders. Harv Rev Psychiatry 2:7–14, 1994

Bourdon KH, Boyd JH, Rae DS, et al: Gender differences in phobias: results of the ECA community survey. J Anxiety Disord 2:227–241, 1988

Breslau N, Davis GC, Andreski P, et al: Sex differences in posttraumatic stress disorder. Arch Gen Psychiatry 54:1044–1048, 1997

Burt VK, Rasgon N: Special considerations in treating bipolar disorder in women. Bipolar Disord 6:2–13, 2004

Castle DJ, Murray RM: The neurodevelopmental basis of sex differences in schizophrenia. Psychol Med 21:565–575, 1991

Centers for Disease Control and Prevention: Physical violence during the 12 months preceding childbirth—Alaska, Maine, Oklahoma, and West Virginia, 1990–1991. MMWR Morb Mortal Wkly Rep 43:132–137, 1994

Choi SH, Kang SB, Joe SH: Changes in premenstrual symptoms in women with schizophrenia: a prospective study. Psychosom Med 6:822–829, 2001

Council of Scientific Affairs, American Medical Association: Violence against women: relevance for medical practitioners. JAMA 267:3184–3189, 1992

Cowell PE, Kostianovsky DJ, Gur RC, et al: Sex differences in neuroanatomical and clinical correlations in schizophrenia. Am J Psychiatry 153:799–805, 1996

Cyr MG, Moulton AW: Substance abuse in women. Obstet Gynecol Clin North Am 17:905–925, 1990

Cyr MG, Moulton AW: The physician's role in prevention, detection, and treatment of alcohol abuse in women. Psychiatr Ann 23:454–462, 1993

Eisenstat SA, Bancroft L: Domestic violence. N Engl J Med 341:886–892, 1999

Ewing JA: Detecting alcoholism: the CAGE questionnaire. JAMA 252:1905–1907, 1984

Flament MF, Rapoport JL: Childhood obsessive-compulsive disorder, in New Findings in Obsessive-Compulsive Disorder. Edited by Insel TR. Washington, DC, American Psychiatric Press, 1984, pp 23–43

Foa EB: Trauma and women: course, predictors, and treatment. J Clin Psychiatry 58(suppl 9):25–28, 1997

Freeman EW, Sammel MD, Liu L, et al: Hormones and menopausal status as predictors of depression in women in transition to menopause. Arch Gen Psychiatry 61:62–70, 2004

Frye MA, Altshuler LL, McElroy SL, et al: Gender differences in prevalence, risk, and clinical correlates of alcoholism comorbidity in bipolar disorder. Am J Psychiatry 160:883–889, 2003

Gossop M, Griffiths P, Powis B, et al: Cocaine: patterns of use, route of administration, and severity of dependence. Br J Psychiatry 164:660–664, 1994

Greenfield SF, Manwani SG, Nargiso JE: Epidemiology of substance use disorders in women. Obstet Gynecol Clin North Am 30:413–446, 2003

Griffin ML, Weiss RD, Mirin SM, et al: A comparison of male and female cocaine abusers. Arch Gen Psychiatry 46:122–126, 1989

Grigoriadis S, Seeman MV: The role of estrogen in schizophrenia: implications for schizophrenia practice guidelines for women. Can J Psychiatry 47:437–442, 2002

Halbreich U: Anxiety disorders in women: a developmental and life-cycle perspective. Depress Anxiety 17:107–110, 2003

Hendrick V, Altshuler LL, Burt VK: Course of psychiatric disorders across the menstrual cycle. Harv Rev Psychiatry 4:200–207, 1996

Hendrick V, Altshuler LL, Gitlin MJ, et al: Gender and bipolar illness. J Clin Psychiatry 61:393–396, 2000

Hoopes SP, Reimherr FW, Hedges DW, et al: Treatment of bulimia nervosa with topiramate in a randomized, double-blind, placebo-controlled trial, part 1: improvement in binge and purge measures. J Clin Psychiatry 64:1335–1341, 2003

Isojarvi JI, Laatikainen TJ, Pakarinen AJ, et al: Polycystic ovaries and hyperandrogenism in women taking valproate for epilepsy. N Engl J Med 329:1383–1388, 1993

Jablensky AV, Morgan V, Zubrick SR, et al: Pregnancy, delivery, and neonatal complications in a population cohort of women with schizophrenia and major affective disorders. Am J Psychiatry 162:79–91, 2005

Jensvold MF, Reed K, Jarrett DB, et al: Menstrual cycle-related depressive symptoms treated with variable antidepressant dosage. J Womens Health 1:109–115, 1992

Kasvikis JG, Tsakiris F, Marks IM: Past history of anorexia nervosa in women with obsessive-compulsive disorder. Int J Eat Disord 5:1069–1075, 1986

Keel PK, Mitchell JE, Miller KB, et al: Long-term outcome of bulimia nervosa. Arch Gen Psychiatry 56:63–69, 1999

Kelly RH, Danielsen BH, Golding JM, et al: Adequacy of prenatal care among women with psychiatric diagnoses giving birth in California in 1994 and 1995. Psychiatr Serv 50:1584–1590, 1999

Kendler KS, Neale MC, Kessler RC, et al: Generalized anxiety disorder in women: a population-based twin study. Arch Gen Psychiatry 49:267–272, 1992

Kendler KS, Neale MC, Kessler RC, et al: Panic disorder in women: a population-based twin study. Psychol Med 23:397–406, 1993

Kendler KS, Thornton LM, Prescott CA: Gender differences in the rates of exposure to stressful life events and sensitivity to their depressogenic effects. Am J Psychiatry 158:587–593, 2001

Kessler RC, McGonagle KA, Swartz M, et al: Sex and depression in the National Comorbidity Survey. I: lifetime prevalence, chronicity and recurrence. J Affect Disord 29:85–96, 1993

Kessler RC, McGonagle KA, Zhao S, et al: Lifetime and 12-month prevalence of DSM-III-R psychiatric disorders in the United States: results from the National Comorbidity Survey. Arch Gen Psychiatry 51:8–19, 1994

Kessler RC, Sonnega A, Bromet E, et al: Posttraumatic stress disorder in the National Comorbidity Survey. Arch Gen Psychiatry 52:1048–1060, 1995

Kornstein SG, Schatzberg AF, Thase ME, et al: Gender differences in treatment response to sertraline versus imipramine in chronic depression. Am J Psychiatry 157:1445–1452, 2000

Kulkarni J, Riedel A, de Castella AR, et al: Estrogen—a potential treatment for schizophrenia. Schizophr Res 48:137–144, 2001

Leach AM: The psychopharmacotherapy of eating disorders. Psychiatr Ann 25:628–633, 1995

Leibenluft E: Women with bipolar illness: clinical and research issues. Am J Psychiatry 153:163–173, 1996

Leibenluft E, Ashman SB, Feldman-Naim S, et al: Lack of relationship between menstrual cycle phase and mood in a sample of women with rapid cycling bipolar disorder. Biol Psychiatry 15:577–580, 1999

Levav I, Kohn R, Golding JM, et al: Vulnerability of Jews to affective disorders. Am J Psychiatry 154:941–947, 1997

Levitan RD, Kaplan AS, Brown GM, et al: Hormonal and subjective responses to intravenous m-chlorophenylpiperazine in women with seasonal affective disorder. Arch Gen Psychiatry 55:244–249, 1998

Lindamer LA, Lohr JB, Harris MJ, et al: Gender-related clinical differences in older patients with schizophrenia. J Clin Psychiatry 60:61–67, 1999

Luef G, Abraham I, Haslinger M, et al: Polycystic ovaries, obesity and insulin resistance in women with epilepsy: a comparative study of carbamazepine and valproic acid in 105 women. J Neurol 249:835–841, 2002

Madden PA, Heath AC, Rosenthal NE, et al: Seasonal changes in mood and behavior: the role of genetic factors. Arch Gen Psychiatry 53:47–55, 1996

Marken PA, Haykal RF, Fisher JN: Management of psychotropic-induced hyperprolactinemia. Clin Pharm 11:851–856, 1992

McIntyre RS, Mancini DA, McCann S, et al: Valproate, bipolar disorder and polycystic ovarian syndrome. Bipolar Disord 5:28–35, 2003

Mickley D: Are you overlooking eating disorders among your patients? Women's Health in Primary Care 3:40–52, 2000

Millman RP: Coping with insomnia: effective drug and non-drug therapies. Women's Health in Primary Care 1:737–745, 1999

Nilsson E, Lichtenstein P, Cnattinguis S, et al: Women with schizophrenia: pregnancy outcome and infant death among their offspring. Schizophr Res 58:221–229, 2002

Nowell PD, Mazumdar S, Buysse DJ, et al: Benzodiazepines and zolpidem for chronic insomnia: a meta-analysis of treatment efficacy. JAMA 278:2170–2177, 1997

Pack AM, Morrell MJ: Epilepsy and bone health in adults. Epilepsy Behav 5 (suppl 2):S24–S29, 2004

Pajer K: New strategies in the treatment of depression in women. J Clin Psychiatry 56 (suppl 2):30–37, 1995

Parker G, Hadzi-Pavlovic D: Is any female preponderance in depression secondary to a primary female preponderance in anxiety disorders? Acta Psychiatr Scand 103:252–256, 2001

Petter LM, Whitehill DL: Management of female sexual assault. Am Fam Physician 58:920–926, 929–930, 1998

Pigott TA: Anxiety disorders in women. Psychiatr Clin North Am 26:621–672, vi–vii, 2003

Polo-Kantola P, Erkkola R, Irjala K, et al: Effect of short-term transdermal estrogen replacement therapy on sleep: a randomized, double-blind crossover trial in postmenopausal women. Fertil Steril 71:873–880, 1999

Quitkin FM, Stewart JW, McGrath PJ, et al: Are there differences between women's and men's antidepressant responses? Am J Psychiatry 159:1848–1854, 2002

Rasgon N: The relationship between polycystic ovary syndrome and antiepileptic drugs: a review of the evidence. J Clin Psychopharmacol. 24:322–334, 2004

Rasgon NL, Altshuler LL, Gudeman D, et al: Medication status and polycystic ovary syndrome in women with bipolar disorder: a preliminary report. J Clin Psychiatry 61:173–178, 2000

Robins LN, Helzer JE, Weissman MM, et al: Lifetime prevalence of specific disorders in three sites. Arch Gen Psychiatry 41:949–958, 1984

Rosenthal NE, Sack DA, Gillin JC, et al: Seasonal affective disorder: a description of the syndrome and preliminary findings with light therapy. Arch Gen Psychiatry 41:72–80, 1984

Rossouw JE, Anderson GL, Prentice RL, et al: Risks and benefits of estrogen plus progestin in healthy postmenopausal women. JAMA 288:321–333, 2002

Sabers A, Buchholt JM, Uldall P, et al: Lamotrigine plasma levels reduced by oral contraceptives. Epilepsy Res 47:151–154, 2001

Schneier FR, Johnson J, Hornig CD, et al: Social phobia: comorbidity and morbidity in an epidemiologic sample. Arch Gen Psychiatry 49:282–288, 1992

Schwartz PJ, Brown C, Wehr TA, et al: Winter seasonal affective disorder: a follow-up study of the first 59 patients of the National Institutes of Mental Health Seasonal Studies Program. Am J Psychiatry 153:1028–1036, 1996

Seeman MV: Interaction of sex, age, and neuroleptic dose. Compr Psychiatry 24:125–128, 1983

Seeman MV: Current outcome in schizophrenia: women vs men. Acta Psychiatr Scand 73:609–617, 1986

Seeman MV: The role of estrogen in schizophrenia. J Psychiatry Neurosci 21:123–127, 1996

Seeman MV: Gender differences in the prescribing of antipsychotic drugs. Am J Psychiatry 161:1324–1333, 2004

Sheikh JI, Leskin GA, Klein DF: Gender differences in panic disorder: findings from the National Comorbidity Survey. Am J Psychiatry 159:55–58, 2002

Silverman JG, Raj A, Mucci LA, et al: Dating violence against adolescent girls and associated substance use, unhealthy weight control, sexual risk behavior, pregnancy, and suicidality. JAMA 286:572–579, 2001

Stewart DE, Boydell KM: Psychological distress during menopause: association across the reproductive life cycle. Int J Psychiatry Med 23:157–162, 1993

Stewart DE, Robinson GE: Violence against women, in American Psychiatric Press Review of Psychiatry, Vol. 14. Edited by Oldham JM, Riba ME. Washington, DC, American Psychiatric Press, 1995, pp 261–285

Szymanski S, Lieberman JA, Alvir JM, et al: Gender differences in onset of illness, treatment response, course, and biologic indexes in first-episode schizophrenic patients. Am J Psychiatry 152:698–703, 1995

Task Force on Panic Anxiety and Its Treatments: Panic anxiety and panic disorder, in Panic Anxiety and Its Treatments: Report of the World Psychiatric Association Presidential Educational Task Force. Edited by Klerman GL, Hirschfield RMA, Weissman MM, et al. Washington, DC, American Psychiatric Press, 1993, pp 3–38

Tondo L, Baldessarini RJ: Rapid cycling in women and men with bipolar manic-depressive disorders. Am J Psychiatry 155:1434–1436, 1998

Vintzileos AM, Ananth CV, Smulian JC, et al: The impact of prenatal care in the United States on preterm births in the presence and absence of antenatal high-risk conditions. Am J Obstet Gynecol 187:1254–1257, 2002a

Vintzileos A, Ananth CV, Smulian JC, et al: The impact of prenatal care on postneonatal deaths in the presence and absence of antenatal high-risk conditions. Am J Obstet Gynecol 187:1258–1262, 2002b

Walsleben JA: Does being female affect one's sleep? J Womens Health Gend Based Med 8:571–572, 1999

Walter H, Gutierrez K, Ramskogler K, et al: Gender-specific differences in alcoholism: implications for treatment. Arch Women Ment Health 6:253–258, 2003

Wehr TA, Goodwin FK: Rapid cycling in manic-depressives induced by tricyclic antidepressants. Arch Gen Psychiatry 36:555–559, 1979

Weissman MM, Leaf PJ, Holzer CE 3rd, et al: The epidemiology of depression: an update on sex differences in rates. J Affect Disord 7:179–188, 1984

Weissman MM, Livingston MB, Leaf PJ, et al: Affective disorders, in Psychiatric Disorders in America: The Epidemiologic Catchment Area Study. Edited by Robins LN, Regier DA. New York, Free Press, 1991, pp 53–80

Wells JE, Bushnell JA, Hornblow AR, et al: Christchurch Psychiatric Epidemiology Study, Part I: methodology and lifetime prevalence for specific psychiatric disorders. Aust N Z J Psychiatry 23:315–326, 1989

Wenger NK, Speroff L, Packard B: Cardiovascular health and disease in women. N Engl J Med 329:247–256, 1993

Winokur G, Coryell W, Akiskal HS, et al: Manic-depressive (bipolar) disorder: the course in light of a prospective ten-year follow-up of 131 patients. Acta Psychiatr Scand 89:102–110, 1994

Wisner KL, Wheeler SB: Prevention of recurrent major postpartum major depression. Hosp Community Psychiatry 45:1191–1196, 1994

Wittchen HU, Essau CA, von Zerssen D, et al: Lifetime and six-month prevalence of mental disorders in the Munich Follow-up Study. Eur Arch Psychiatry Clin Neurosci 241:247–258, 1992

Wohlfarth T, Storosum JG, Elferink AJ, et al. Response to tricyclic antidepressants: independent of gender? Am J Psychiatry 161: 370–372, 2004

Yehuda R: Post-traumatic stress disorder. New Engl J Medicine. 346:108–114, 2002

Yonkers KA: The association between premenstrual dysphoric disorder and other mood disorders. J Clin Psychiatr 58 (suppl 15):19–25, 1997

Yonkers KA, Gurguis G: Gender differences in the prevalence and expression of anxiety disorders, in Gender and Psychopathology. Edited by Seeman MV. Washington, DC, American Psychiatric Press, 1995, pp 113–130

Yonkers KA, Zlotnick C, Allsworth J, et al: Is the course of panic disorder the same in women and men? Am J Psychiatry 155:596–602, 1998

Zerbe KJ: Anxiety disorders in women. Bull Menninger Clin 59 (2 suppl A):A38–A52, 1995

# 10

# Female-Specific Cancers

## Breast Cancer

One of nine women will have breast cancer in their lifetimes (Rowland and Holland 1990), making it the most prevalent of all cancers in women. The disease is rare in women under age 30 years; the rate rises among women in their early 40s, stabilizes, and then increases again in women older than age 55 years. Two-thirds of all breast cancer patients are older than age 50 years. Women with certain risk factors (Table 10–1), particularly a first-degree relative with breast cancer, tend to feel even more anxious about their likelihood of developing the disease. A study of women with breast cancer found that emotional, sexual, and social functioning tends to be better 2–5 years after initial treatment, compared to immediately after treatment and after 5 years (Holzner et al. 2001). This finding suggests that women with breast cancer experience impaired quality of life long after treatment.

The stress of receiving a diagnosis of breast cancer and of undergoing treatment is compounded by worry about disfigurement. Over the past

**Table 10–1.    Risk factors for breast cancer**

Family history, especially in first-degree female relatives

First pregnancy after age 30 years

Nulliparity

Early menarche

Late menopause

Increasing age

Caucasian race

Obesity

Higher socioeconomic status

History of benign breast disease

Previous carcinoma in one breast, especially in premenopausal women

Nicotine use

Alcohol use

Use of exogenous hormones (controversial)

20 years, however, breast-sparing procedures have increasingly replaced radical mastectomies, dramatically reducing the effect on the woman's physical appearance after surgery. Although breast-conserving surgery has a beneficial effect on self-image and self-esteem, women who receive this treatment may feel greater uncertainty about their long-term survival (Rowland and Holland 1990). However, research suggests that breast-sparing procedures have outcomes equally favorable to those of radical mastectomies (Rowland and Holland 1990).

The treatment strategies for breast cancer are surgery, radiation therapy, and chemotherapy. Surgical procedures include radical mastectomy (removal of the breast, the chest muscles, and the underarm lymph nodes), modified radical mastectomy (removal of the breast, the underarm lymph nodes, and the lining over the chest muscles), total (simple) mastectomy (removal of only the breast), partial (segmental) mastectomy (removal of the tumor and some surrounding tissue), and lumpectomy (removal of only the tumor; it is followed by radiation therapy). Radiation therapy may also be used after segmental or total mastectomy, particularly if cancer has been found in the lymph nodes.

Adjuvant chemotherapy sometimes follows the surgery and employs agents that may include cyclophosphamide, methotrexate, 5-fluorouracil, and doxorubicin. For women with estrogen-receptor positive tumors, hormonal therapy with tamoxifen may be used. Recent data suggest that aromatase inhibitors, such as letrozole, may extend disease-free survival after completion of a standard regimen of tamoxifen (Goss et al. 2003). Monoclonal antibody therapy is also available to treat breast cancer in some patients. After mastectomy, breast reconstruction is an option that may significantly enhance a woman's sense of sexuality and self-esteem.

# Gynecological Cancer

Gynecological cancers produce significant stress, not only because they are life-threatening but also because they affect organs associated with reproduction, sexuality, and femininity. In order of frequency, gynecological cancers affect the cervix, endometrium, ovary, vagina, and vulva. Ovarian cancer, however, produces the greatest mortality rate. Surgical treatments for gynecological cancers include hysterectomy (removal of the uterus), ovariectomy (removal of the ovaries), vulvectomy (excision of the external genitalia), and pelvic exenteration (a more radical surgical procedure involving removal of the bladder, vagina, uterus, and rectum). Chemotherapeutic agents may be initiated after surgery and usually include vincristine, vinblastine, and interferon. After pelvic exenteration or vulvectomy, construction of a neovagina helps restore some sexual function.

For women with gynecologic malignancies, quality of life is most adversely affected from the time of diagnosis through completion of treatment. Quality of life tends to improve over the year after treatment and then remains fairly stable. Risk factors for poor quality of life include treatment with radiotherapy or more than one mode of treatment, increased length of treatment, and younger age. Patients who cope by disengaging from their caregivers or by avoiding problems are more likely to experience depression and tend to have more difficulty functioning. Lower levels of education, lower levels of spiritual and religious beliefs, and lack of help at home are also risk factors for poor quality of life in gynecologic cancer patients (Pearman 2003).

Sexual problems after treatment may result from the physical effects of surgery or pelvic irradiation. Psychological issues associated with the cancer, which may also influence a woman's sexuality, include a fear of recurrence of cancer and a decreased sense of femininity from loss of the uterus or other pelvic organs. The partner's attitude toward a woman's diagnosis and treatment also affects her sexuality. The partner's sexual interest after the surgery helps maintain a woman's sexual functioning (McCartney 1993).

# Psychiatric Consultation

A psychiatric consultation may be requested for a woman undergoing treatment for breast or gynecological cancer. In addition to conducting a standard psychiatric assessment, the psychiatrist should address issues that are particularly relevant to this population, including depression and anxiety, interpersonal issues, and common fears and concerns.

## Depression and Anxiety

A patient's physicians and family may dismiss her depressive symptoms as normal reactions to an illness and may attribute physical problems (poor appetite, fatigue, loss of sexual desire) to the illness and its treatment rather than to a mood disorder. A careful psychiatric assessment is therefore necessary. Although most women who receive a diagnosis of breast cancer appear to cope relatively well, between one-quarter and one-third experience significant emotional distress and depression (Rowland 1999). Risk factors for depression in breast cancer patients include having a history of depression, having advanced cancer, being in significant pain, or being younger than age 50 years at the time of the initial diagnosis (Rowland et al. 1999; Massie and Holland 1990). A woman's coping style also influences her emotional state during treatment: a sense of helplessness and fatalism, in contrast to a sense of control over events, produces greater psychological morbidity (Watson et al. 1991). Organic etiologies for mood disorders in cancer patients include the depressive side effects of steroids and some chemotherapeutic agents (Table 10–2). It is not unusual for a woman to experience depression and anxiety once she ends her course of chemotherapy, as she may have come to view the chemotherapy as a protection against progression of the cancer (Hamilton 1999).

Psychiatric treatment strategies include supportive therapy and cognitive approaches to reduce the patient's sense of helplessness. Education about the treatment can increase a woman's sense of control and of the predictability of

**Table 10–2.**   Anticancer drugs associated with psychiatric side effects

| Drug | Side effect | | | |
| --- | --- | --- | --- | --- |
| | **Delirium** | **Depression** | **Anxiety** | **Psychosis** |
| Cisplatin | X | – | – | – |
| Cyclophosphamide | X | – | – | – |
| Dacarbazine | – | – | X | – |
| Hexamethylmelamine | X | X | – | – |
| Methotrexate | X | – | – | – |
| 5-Fluorouracil | X | – | – | – |
| Vincristine | X | X | – | X |
| Vinblastine | X | X | X | – |
| Interferon | X | X | – | – |
| Corticosteroids | X | – | – | X |
| Tamoxifen | X | – | – | X (one report) |

*Note.*   – = side effect is not present.
*Source.*   Derived from McCartney 1993 and Ron et al. 1992.

the situation. Group therapy is a very useful modality for women with cancer. The literature regarding whether group therapy actually prolongs survival is contradictory (Goodwin et al. 2001; Spiegel et al. 1989). However, although supportive-expressive group therapy in patients with metastatic breast cancer does not appear to extend survival, it does improve mood and the perception of pain, particularly in women who initially experience great distress (Goodwin et al. 2001)

By enhancing appetite and sleep, antidepressant medications may be helpful not only for mood but also for a patient's physical condition. Tricyclic antidepressants (TCAs) have the additional advantage of reducing pain. On the other hand, less sedating antidepressants may be preferable for patients experiencing lethargy or undergoing radiation therapy, a procedure associated with significant fatigue. There is a case report of tamoxifen-associated reduction in serum TCA and metabolite levels (Jefferson 1995). For antidepressant-treated patients who are taking tamoxifen or other medications that interact with the cytochrome P450 system, it may be useful to check serum levels of parent and metabolite compounds and to raise the dose when clinically indicated.

Anxiety may be treated with cognitive-behavioral strategies (e.g., guided imagery, progressive relaxation) and with low doses of anxiolytic medications. For patients with initial insomnia secondary to anxiety, short-acting benzodiazepines such as oxazepam or temazepam may be useful for several weeks. Low doses of trazodone (e.g., 50–100 mg/night) may also be helpful.

Patients should be counseled regarding sleep hygiene and avoidance of caffeine and alcohol. Women with cancer who have a history of heavy alcohol use may increase their alcohol intake and risk alcohol abuse or dependence. These women should be encouraged to share their concerns and fears with nonjudgmental professionals or lay persons (including Alcoholics Anonymous sponsors). These helping persons can assist the patient with the reality of cancer and adapting to the illness.

## Interpersonal Issues

The diagnosis and treatment of breast or gynecological cancer may have a significant effect on the woman's marital or sexual relationship. A woman's sense of sexuality and femininity may be reduced after surgery, particularly if the surgery was extensive. The pain of past sexual traumas may be revived during gynecological cancer treatment. Induced menopause from radical hysterectomy often precipitates hot flashes, cold sweats, and disturbed sleep, which frequently cannot be treated with hormone replacement therapy because it is contraindicated for patients with certain kinds of breast or gynecological cancers. Continued sleep deprivation may escalate into depression, irritability, and anxiety.

A woman's partner may fear hurting the woman by resuming sexual activity or may want to avoid seeing her surgical scars, which are a reminder of her illness and mortality. It may be helpful for a partner to be involved in the treatment decisions and to help with dressings and other postsurgical care. Conjoint education and supportive therapy are often beneficial as the couple deals with interpersonal issues and the resumption of sexual activity. Special consideration should be given to couples with a history of conflict or poor communication, because they are at greater risk for poor adjustment.

The availability of other interpersonal supports should be explored. Psychological intervention with a patient's family may enhance a sense of family unity and support. The Reach to Recovery program provides peer counseling, matching women who have had surgery for breast cancer with women who are facing it. Group therapy, offered by hospital-based cancer centers and local branches of the American Cancer Society, provides both psychological and practical support for the patient and family (see Appendix).

## Common Fears and Concerns

It is natural for a patient to have concerns about disfigurement, recurrence, pain, and death. Anxiety about the diagnosis may result in a delay in obtaining appropriate care. The patient may also fear that medical and surgical interventions will produce permanent sexual dysfunction and will render her unattractive to her partner. She may also worry about the welfare of her children while she is in the hospital or in the event of her death. The psychiatrist may be particularly helpful in exploring the patient's fears and expectations and in acting as a liaison with the oncology team to ensure that the patient obtains adequate management of pain and nausea and that she is informed about her treatment course, options, and prognosis. Negative psychiatric side effects of chemotherapy should be assessed and managed with the aid of psychiatric consultation and follow-up. Interventions addressing practical issues, such as child care and financial concerns, can significantly reduce a patient's anxiety while she undergoes treatment. The patient should also be reassured that all possible therapeutic measures have been employed, particularly if her cancer is terminal, because this information may help her accept the cancer.

# References

Goodwin PJ, Leszcz M, Ennis M, et al: The effect of group psychosocial support on survival in metastatic breast cancer. New Engl J Med 345:1719–1726, 2001

Goss PE, Ingle JM, Martino S, et al: A randomized trial of letrozole in postmenopausal women after five years of tamoxifen therapy for early-stage breast cancer. New Engl J Med 349:1793–1802, 2003

Hamilton AB: Psychological aspects of ovarian cancer. Cancer Invest 17:335–341, 1999

Holzner B, Kemmler G, Kopp M, et al: Quality of life in breast cancer patients—not enough attention for long-term survivors? Psychosomatics 42:117–123, 2001

Jefferson JW: Tamoxifen-associated reduction in tricyclic antidepressant levels in blood (letter). J Clin Psychopharmacol 15:223–224, 1995

Massie MJ, Holland JC: Depression and the cancer patient. J Clin Psychiatry 51 (suppl):12–17, 1990

McCartney CF: Gynecologic oncology, in Psychological Aspects of Women's Health Care. Edited by Stewart DE, Stotland NL. Washington, DC, American Psychiatric Press, 1993, pp 291–312

Pearman T: Quality of life and psychosocial adjustment in gynecologic cancer survivors. Health Qual Life Outcomes 1:33–39, 2003

Ron IG, Inbar MJ, Barak Y, et al: Organic delusional syndrome associated with tamoxifen treatment. Cancer 69:1415–1417, 1992

Rowland JH: Anxiety and the blues after breast cancer: how common are they? CNS Spectr 4:40–54, 1999

Rowland JH, Holland JC: Breast cancer, in Handbook of Psychooncology: Psychological Care of the Patient With Cancer. Edited by Holland JC, Rowland JH. New York, Oxford University Press, 1990, pp 188–207

Spiegel D, Bloom JR, Kraemer HC, et al: Effect of psychosocial treatment on survival of patients with metastatic breast cancer. Lancet 2:888–891, 1989

Watson M, Greer S, Rowden L, et al: Relationships between emotional control, adjustment to cancer and depression and anxiety in breast cancer patients. Psychol Med 21:51–57, 1991

# Resources and Support Groups

## Women's Issues

The National Women's Health Information Center, U.S. Department of Health and Human Services; 800-994-9662; http://www.4women.gov. Provides information for women on a variety of topics, including heart disease, disabilities, pregnancy, breast-feeding, HIV/AIDS, etc.

American College of Obstetricians and Gynecologists, 409 12th Street SW, Washington, DC 20090-6920; 202-638-5577; http://www.acog.org. Professional organization of obstetricians and gynecologists. Provides information on a variety of topics of interest to women, including abortion, contraception, pregnancy, birth, postpartum, breast-feeding, menopause, female-specific cancers, premenstrual syndrome, etc.

## Contraception

Association of Reproductive Health Professionals, 2401 Pennsylvania Avenue NW, Suite 350, Washington, DC 20037-1730; 202-466-3825; http://www.arhp.org/patienteducation/interactivetools. International nonprofit association of health care providers, researchers, and educators. Offers interactive questionnaire that guides patient in making contraceptive decisions.

Planned Parenthood Federation of America, 434 West 33rd Street, New York, NY 10001-2601, 800-230-7526; http://www.ppfa.org. Provides information about pregnancy options, birth control, emergency contraception, abortion, adoption, parenting, pregnancy, and sexual health.

## Infertility

RESOLVE: The National Infertility Association, 1310 Broadway, Somerville, MA 02144-1731; 617-623-0744; http://www.resolve.org. National self-help organization for infertile couples. Sponsors support groups throughout the country to destigmatize the issue of infertility and enable couples to feel strengthened and less isolated. Telephone help line (888-623-0744) operates 9:00 A.M.–12:00 noon and 1:00–4:00 P.M. eastern time, Monday and Wednesday through Friday; 9:00 A.M.–12:00 noon and 1:00–9:00 P.M. eastern time, on Tuesday. Memberships available. Send self-addressed, stamped envelope for further information.

## Pregnancy and Postpartum Disorders

Postpartum Support International, 927 N. Kellogg Avenue, Santa Barbara, CA 93111-1022; 805-967-7636; http://www.postpartum.net. An international network of individuals and organizations whose purpose is to increase awareness among public and professional communities about the emotional changes women often experience during pregnancy and after the birth of a baby. Provides referrals for group therapy, individual therapists, and psychiatrists to women with postpartum depression.

Motherisk; 416-813-6780; http://www.motherisk.org. Canadian-based organization that provides information on morning sickness, safety or risks of drugs in pregnancy and lactation, alcohol and other substance use in pregnancy, HIV/AIDS in pregnancy. Hotlines:

Alcohol and Substance Use Helpline: 877-327-4636

Nausea and Vomiting of Pregnancy Helpline: 800-436-8477

HIV and HIV Treatment in Pregnancy: 888-246-5840

Massachusetts General Hospital Center for Women's Mental Health; http://www.womensmentalhealth.org/. Web site of the Massachusetts General Hospital Reproductive Psychiatry Resource and Information Center. Discusses psychiatric conditions in women, including premenstrual syndrome, postpartum depression, and perimenopausal mood changes.

La Leche League International; 1400 N. Meacham Road, Schaumburg, IL 60173-4808; 800-LALECHE (800-525-3243); http://www.lalecheleague.org. Organization that promotes breast-feeding and provides information and support for new mothers.

## Menopause and Hormone Therapy

North American Menopause Society (NAMS), P.O. Box 94527, Cleveland, OH 44101-4527; 800-774-5342; http://www.menopause.org. Nonprofit organization promoting women's health during midlife and beyond through an understanding of menopause. Provides information on all aspects of menopause.

American Association of Retired Persons, 601 E Street NW, Washington, DC 20049-2208; 888-OUR-AARP (888-687-2277); http://www.aarp.org. Large advocacy organization that supports the health, economic, and social needs of women and men age 55 years and older.

## Eating Disorders

National Eating Disorders Association, 603 Stewart Street, Suite 803, Seattle, WA 98101-1264; 206-382-3587; http://www.edap.org. Nonprofit organization to prevent eating disorders and provide treatment referrals to patients with anorexia, bulimia, and binge-eating disorder and those concerned with body image and weight issues.

## Domestic Violence

National Domestic Violence Hotline; 800-799-7233; http://www.ndvh.org. Information about domestic violence and the names and telephone numbers of local shelters for victims of domestic violence.

## Alcohol and Drug Abuse

National Institute on Drug Abuse (NIDA); http://www.nida.nih.gov/WHGD/WHGDHome.html. Lists NIDA news releases and publications relevant to drug and alcohol abuse disorders in women.

## Cancer

National Cancer Institute, Cancer Information Service; 800-4-CANCER (800-422-6237). Hotline for information on treatments and psychosocial resources.

Cancervive, 11636 Chayote Street, Los Angeles, CA 90049-3308; 310-203-9232; http://cancervive.org. Group and individual counseling for women who are at least 6 months posttreatment. Newsletter publication.

The National Coalition for Cancer Survivorship, 1010 Wayne Avenue, Suite 770, Silver Spring, MD 20910-5634; 877-622-7937. National network of independent groups and individuals dedicated to providing support for cancer patients and their families.

Reach to Recovery: A Program of the American Cancer Society; 800-227-2345; http://www.cancer.org. Women who have had breast surgery (mastectomies with and without breast reconstruction or lumpectomies) visit and counsel women before and after their surgery. Provides patients, family, and friends with information about cancer, decision tools, clinical trials, and ways to cope with cancer.

We Can Weekend, American Cancer Society; 800-227-2345; http://www.cancer.org. Retreats for families dealing with cancer. Focus is on problems encountered by families affected by cancer. Designed for families with children and adolescents. Offered in many locations around the United States.

Y-ME National Breast Cancer Organization, 212 West Van Buren, Suite 1000, Chicago, IL 60607-3908; http://www.y-me.org; national toll-free hotline: 800-221-2141, 9:00 A.M.–5:00 P.M. central time; 24-hour telephone: 312-986-8338. Trained volunteers, most of them breast cancer survivors, provide information and support.

Abramson Cancer Center of the University of Pennsylvania; http://www.oncolink.upenn.edu/. Provides information about cancer, treatment options, clinical trials, cancer resources, and literature.

# Index

*Page numbers printed in **boldface** type refer to tables or figures.*